A GUIDED TOUR THROUGH THE HUMAN ANATOMY

THE DIFFERENT BODY SYSTEMS IN HUMANS

FUNCTIONAL HEALTH SERIES

SAM FURY

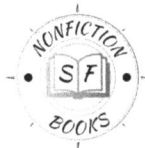

WARNINGS AND DISCLAIMERS

The information in this publication is made public for reference only.

Neither the author, publisher, nor anyone else involved in the production of this publication is responsible for how the reader uses the information or the result of his/her actions.

CONTENTS

THANKS FOR YOUR PURCHASE

Get Your Next SF Nonfiction Book FREE!

Claim the book of your choice at:

www.SFNonfictionBooks.com

You will also be among the first to know of all the latest releases, discount offers, bonus content, and more.

Go to:

www.SFNonfictionBooks.com

Thanks again for your support.

INTRODUCTION

One of the most interesting subjects to study is the human body. Why? In most ways, you're learning about yourself. You're learning about all the different body parts and functions that come together to make you a functional being, and in many ways, this is both amazing and exciting. Perhaps you've watched a cut heal or seen the miracle of birth and were amazed by how it all works together to ensure life. If you've ever wondered about some of it and desired to understand the human body without a complex maze of peer-reviewed articles and textbooks, then you're in the right place.

Human anatomy research has a rich past that goes back to the earliest civilizations. Among the first people to document anatomical observations were the Egyptians through their mummification practices. Greek doctors like Hippocrates and Galen made important contributions with Galen's work remaining a major reference for centuries. Then the Renaissance period saw an emergence of figures such as Andreas Vesalius, whose precise dissections and illustrations significantly altered our view of human anatomy. Today, technology has enabled us to investigate the body in ways our predecessors could only dream of.

So, in helping you to understand the mysteries and wonders involved, I'll be your guide through this discovery of your very own body—and not your ordinary guide. Together, we'll break down otherwise complicated information into simple and engaging concepts so that, by the end of this book, you'll not only be more knowledgeable about your own anatomy but also gain a deeper appreciation for the incredible machine that keeps you going.

From our bones that provide structure to our muscles that support movement and our nerves that send signals to the blood, you'll soon come to know every part of the human body's unique and important role. Fully understanding the functions of these systems can enhance your life and how you interact with your body. For example, it can help you to make more informed health decisions, identify potential issues you may have, and provide better care for others.

Each chapter of this book will act as a different stop along a guided tour, kind of like in the 2001 American live-action and animated film, *Osmosis Jones* with Bill Murray and Chris Rock. Use your imagination as we tour the body and enjoy the experience, whether we're exploring the confines of the skull or the tips of the toes, don't be afraid. Before we begin, let's review some of the highlights to come on our journey.

First Stop: The Skeletal System

We'll then get right into it with the very framework of our existence: the skeletal system. This system is much more than what you remember from middle school or high school. That is an active structure that supports and protects organs, directs our muscles and helps us move like well-oiled machines. Can you imagine life without bones? We'd all be a blob, something out of a sci-fi or horror movie.

Thankfully, bones exist, and we'll be able to explore the different types of bones, from the long bones in our legs—like the shin bone that really hurts when you hit it—to the flat bones in our skull, our personal security guards. You'll understand how they grow, repair, and sometimes break if you're not too careful. You'll also learn about joints, the connections that give us flexibility and movement, and examine common bone-related disorders and how we can maintain bone health.

Second Stop: The Muscular System

Next, we'll step into the powerhouse that is behind every action you've ever taken. Imagine playing Red Light, Green Light, but you never got the green light to move and always had to stay in place. Muscles are like our body's green light, allowing us to move, and they're used more often than we know. In fact, they're necessary for everything. From reading the words of this book to turning these pages, muscles help us perform every-day activities. So, during this stop we'll break down the three types of muscles—skeletal, smooth, and cardiac—and see how they work, grow, and unfortunately suffer from injuries or diseases at times. Understanding muscle anatomy will also give you insights into fitness and physical health, helping you learn how you can stay active and strong.

Third Stop: The Nervous System

Our tour will continue with the nervous system, the body's control center. Think about all the cables and cords that come along with a router and modem; they might seem complicated, but they all have a specific purpose. This is what the nervous system is like: a complex network of wires that send signals all over the body. We'll venture into the brain—your command center—and to the spinal cord, the main hubs, and the peripheral nerves. For example, you will learn how neurons transmit signals and what happens when things go wrong, which can lead to conditions like Alzheimer's or multiple sclerosis. I promise to make it easy for you though.

Fourth Stop: The Circulatory System

The circulatory system, the body's transportation network, would be up next. This system is like the best transportation service in town; it's focused on moving blood, which in turn carries oxygen and nutrients to every cell. You'll want to be on this train because it'll take you all the way to the heart, which, for most of us, has been working since your days in the womb. It takes no day off! You'll also come to know the wide network of blood vessels that act like tree branches distributing blood all throughout our bodies. Don't you just want to know about heart health, high blood pressure (hypertension), low blood pressure (hypotension), and common cardiovascular problems? They might sound daunting, but I can say from experience that they're not as boring as they sound!

Fifth Stop: The Respiratory System

Ahhh! There's nothing quite like fresh air, literally! Breathing is an unconscious act which we do every second; none of us can survive without breathing. Whether you're up in space headed to Mars or the moon, or down below on the ocean bed doing research, if we are to survive, oxygen is a key component. So, in our visit to the respiratory system, get ready to cover everything from the nose to the lungs. You'll learn how and why we breathe in oxygen and breathe out carbon dioxide; you'll also learn the mechanics of breathing, how the gases exchange, and the job of respiratory system to keep everything balanced and stable. We'll additionally touch on some commonly known respiratory conditions such as asthma and ways of promoting sound lung health.

Sixth Stop: The Digestive System

But now for one of the most exciting stops: the digestive system. Everyone loves food, but what really happens after you take a bite? It's not something you can just look at with a mirror at or even feel to some extent. The digestive system is truly a marvelous thing because it takes apart food into substances that our body can use. So, just like the last thing you ate, let's put on our safety belts and go for a roller-coaster ride along the digestive system, starting from the mouth to the intestines.

Seventh Stop: The Urinary System

The next stop you may want to avoid, but unfortunately its a one-way tour. It's imperative that we visit the urinary system. It may not seem like a great place to stop on your journey, but this system is important for waste removal and maintaining fluid balance. We shall take a deep look inside the kidneys, which are filtration power-houses, and find out how urine moves from them to bladder. What a ride! You'll learn about kidney health, common problems such as urinary tract infections (UTIs) and kidney stones, and the means by which they might be avoided.

Eight Stop: The Endocrine System

Most of our bodily functions are regulated through hormones like that moderate our growth, metabolism and mood. In other words, when we study endocrine system more thoroughly, we will learn about its main glands that release various hormones in the body. You will also be enlightened about how hormonal imbalances affect your health along with some solutions to keep hormone levels under control.

Ninth Stop: The Lymphatic and Immune Systems

The body's defense mechanisms are simply amazing. It may not look like it when you see it outside, but inside there is so much defending going on against many forms of threats. So, we'll be learning about this by visiting lymphatic system, which helps us keep off infections. We'll also make it a double stop and visit the the immune system, our front line of defense. Understanding these systems can help you appreciate how we fight off diseases and what happens when the immune system malfunctions.

Final Stop: The Reproductive System

Finally, our tour will conclude with reproductive system visitation. Among other things, the reproductive system is one of your most valuable assets because it plays a role in new life formation within you. We'll discuss male and female reproductive systems' anatomy and function as well as how they collaborate in order to maintain humanity's continued existence.

So, let's get going. Your one-of-a-kind tour awaits!

THE SKELETAL SYSTEM

The bones, joints, and connective tissues that make up the skeletal system are very impressive to behold. They're like the scaffolding of a large structure, carefully constructed to provide strength and adaptability. According to Italian anatomist Niccolò Massa, as outlined in The History of the Skeleton (2019):

> It is very clearly apparent from the admonitions of Galen how great is the usefulness of a knowledge of the bones, since the bones are the foundation of the rest of the parts of the body and all the members rest upon them and are supported, as proceeding from a primary base. Thus if anyone is ignorant of the structure of the bones it follows necessarily that he will be ignorant of very many other things along with them.

Structure and Function

Each of the 206 bones in an adult's body has a different function. Each bone type has its own design necessary for the skeletal system' to keep the body moving, protect it, and support its physiological processes. It's really amazing how different bone structures and functions are, ranging from the strong femur located in your thigh to the tiny bones in your hands and feet. This diversity ensures that the skeletal system performs its different roles efficiently.

For example, protective bones like those in the cranium—also called the skull—ought to be sturdy and curved, as this helps to shield the brain against any collision. On the other hand, bones used for movement such as those found on limbs should combine strength with flexibility to allow for many movements without breaking.

Meanwhile, different functional requirements are reflected in varying densities and compositions of bones. Compact and dense bones provide rigidity required for weight bearing and support, whereas spongy porous bones often exist where they will experience compressions and thus help absorb shocks reducing the overall weight of the skeleton. Thus, this sophisticated design of the skeletal system and the specialization of each bone allow for maintaining a frame around our bodies that also supports our bodies internally, protects important organs, assists when we move around, and contributes to homeostasis, making this biological engineering a wonder within ourselves.

Overview of Bones and Their Functions

To understand the human skeletal system, it is important to start by examining the bones from a closer perspective. Bones are rigid structures. Each adapts uniquely to fulfill specific roles regarding our well-being and movement. They form the framework that supports our bodies, allowing us to stand up, move around, and interact with our surroundings. However, there are several other functions of bones, apart from providing support:

Protection

Our bones safeguard our inner body organs. The brain is housed within the skull, the heart and lungs are placed inside the ribcage, and the vertebral column protects the spinal cord against any potential damage. This coordination of all our bones to perform their functions provides overall protection and ensures our survival. Without this coverage, these essential organs would be vulnerable to injury from even minor accidents or falls.

Movement

Bones also act as levers that muscles pull on to create movement. The interplay between bones and muscles enables us to walk, run, pick things up, and much more than we often realize. Given that bones are rigid, it is our joints—where bones meet—that facilitate different forms of movement. Whether it's simply moving your finger to pick a piece of thread off the carpet or engaging in professional ice-skating, our bones and joints are working together to support movement.

Mineral Storage

Calcium and phosphorus are some of the vital minerals stored within bones primarily for emergencies. These minerals might be required for the maintenance of various bodily functions, such as nerve transmission, muscle activity or blood clotting.

Blood Cell Production

Blood cells, including red blood cells that transport oxygen throughout the body, are mainly created in the bone marrow within certain bones. The bone marrow also includes white blood cells, responsible for combating disease-causing organisms, and platelets that aid in clotting.

Energy Storage

Finally, bones also store lipids, a group of naturally occurring molecules including fats, oils, and waxes. They are important for storing energy and are found in the yellow marrow of the bone.

Types of Bones

Bones typically vary in shape and size according to their specific functions. Our bodies would face significant functional challenges if all our bones were the same size and density. The intricate balance and specialization which our varied bone structures offer would be lost. For instance, the dexterity and precision required in tasks like writing or grasping objects would be diminished if we had huge, dense bones in areas such as hands and feet. Conversely, a lack of enough support would mean that having small, less dense bones in our weight bearing regions like the spine and legs could result in more frequent fractures, making it impossible for the bones to support the body weight adequately and leading to impaired movement. This is why we have different types of bones. Let's take a look at the four major types of bones:

Long Bones

These are narrow, longer bones, and are predominantly located in limbs. Some instances include the thigh bone, called femur, along with the humerus or upper arm bone, and shinbone, called tibia. Long bones are of utmost importance when it comes to movement and bear most of the body's weight.

Short Bones

These bones have equal width and length, giving them stability as well as limited range of motion. They mainly occur in wrists and ankles. Examples include carpals or wrist bones as well as tarsals/ankle bones. Short bones play a role in shock absorption because they help disperse forces.

Flat Bones

These ones tend to be thin, flat, sometimes curved with great protective coverage; they also act like muscle attachment points. The sternum (breastbone), scapulae (shoulder blades), and cranial bones have this type of bone structure. Flat bones have large roles to play, such as protecting internal organs by acting like shields or guards while providing surfaces for muscular attachment.

Irregular Bones

Just like the name suggests, this type of bone does not conform to any particular form. Its complex shapes set it apart from the rest. Examples include our vertebrae/spinal column and many facial bones, among others. Irregular bones perform specialized functions, including protecting nervous tissue, allowing for multiple points of articulation with other skeletal parts, especially at joints that require flexibility, and maintaining its primary role within the organism's structure.

Bone Structure

one structure is also varying and complex. It mostly consists of two types of tissues: compact and spongy bone.

Compact Bone

This is a hard and rigid outer layer of bone that withstands body weight and mechanical tension. Osteons, referred to as Haversian systems, are the core skeletal system building blocks that make up compact bones. Concentric rings of calcified matrix (the hardened part of bones that give them strength enclose a canal which is home to blood vessels and nerves in each osteon.

Spongy Bone

This is also referred to as cancellous bone. This tissue is found inside bones where it forms a porous honeycomb appearance. Spongy bones have less density than compact bones and thus contribute to the skeleton's overall lighter weight. Where blood cell formation occurs in cancellous or spongy bone, the red bone marrow fills in the gaps.

Numerous cells that support bone formation, maintenance, and repair are also present in bones.

Osteoblasts

These cells are responsible for bone formation. They make the bone's structure and substance and play a role in the mineralization process. Osteoblasts also play an essential role in healing fractures and the growth of new bones.

Osteocytes

These are mature bone cells that maintain the bone matrix. They originate from osteoblasts and position themselves within it more specifically helping to regulate mineral content while communicating with others.

Osteoclasts

These cells break down the hard bony tissue involved in maintaining calcium level for developmental processes taking place in other parts of body.

Bone Remodeling

This is a continuous process involving the osteoclasts and osteoblasts. It is aimed at renewing worn out or injured parts within the bone. By allowing adaptation to new stressors, repair to minor damages, as well as maintaining minerals balance, they enable survival from youth to old age. This bone remodeling function targets any damaged part by replacing it with healthy, new tissues, thus making them fit again.

Major Bones and Joints

Bones are living tissues which constantly regenerate themselves. They store vital minerals like calcium and phosphorus, supply them to the bloodstream when needed, and contain bone marrow, which is where new blood cells are made. This ever-changing system is necessary for maintaining the homeostasis—the balance of our body.

Meanwhile, joints serve as links between skeletal points, allowing for various movements to take place. They come in several different forms, including hinge joints (elbows or knees) or socket-and-ball joints (shoulders or hips). Actions from simply walking to advanced dancing can be facilitated by these kinds of articulations.

Major Bones

To have a thorough understanding of how the skeletal framework facilitates your daily pursuits, it is important to know some major bones in the body and their functions.

Skull

The skull, though from outside it may feel like one round, hard shell, is made up of many bones. These bones form our facial structure and provide a protective covering for our thinking box, the brain. Some of the incidents the skull and facial bones protect us from are injuries to the brain from due to collision or fall. Sure, a helmet goes a long way, but so do our skull and facial bones. The complex structure of the cranium also permits the attachment of the muscles responsible for our chewing muscles and facial expressions like frowning and smiling.

Spine

The vertebral column, also called the spine, consists of individual bones called vertebrae running from base of skull to pelvis area. It encloses the spinal cord, supports the head, and has ribs and muscles attached to it. Spinal curvature—the natural, gentle curves in the spine—aids in weight distribution across the body and in balancing activities. It is divided into five regions, namely: cervical, thoracic, lumbar, sacral, and coccygeal vertebrae with each having distinct characteristics and roles. Some examples of these roles is the way the cervical vertebrae allows for a wide range head movements while the lumbar supports body weight.

Ribs

There are 12 pairs of ribs that attach from behind to spine around to the sternum—also called the breastbone—in front, forming the rib cage. These protect the heart and lungs as well support the upper part of the body. Joints between our ribs allow for breathing movement by enlarging when we inhale air. Each rib pair connects posteriorly with the spine while anteriorly they either join the breast-bone directly or through costal cartilages—flexible connective tissues —which gives them a bit of flexibility for movement and impact absorption.

Pelvis

The pelvis is shaped like a basin and bears the weight of the upper body and links lower limbs to joints. It provides a solid base for standing and walking and safeguards the reproductive organs. The hip bones, sacrum, and coccyx make up the pelvis. Weight is distributed evenly between the upper and lower limbs, thanks to the design of the pelvis, and there are attachment places for muscles that allow for posture and movement.

Limbs

These bones include the lower limb's tibia, fibula and femur in the lower limb and the upper limb's humerus, ulna and radius. These lengthy bones support weight for a variety of physical activities and are essential for movement. The femur, which happens to be the longest bone in the body, supports an upright stance, including while walking and running. Meanwhile, the shoulder girdle is where arm's bones are connected, while the pelvic girdle connects the legs and enables flexing, movement, and strength.

Major Joints

Joints are our body's amazing parts that allow us to move and be flexible. Because every kind of joint is made differently to enable certain movements, our mobility and functionality are guaranteed. Together, these joints enable a variety of actions, from simple daily chores to intricate muscular movements. Let's zero in for a bit on some of our major joints.

Ball-and-Socket Joints

These joints, such as those in our shoulders and hips, have a great deal of motion in different directions. They make motions like arm swings and leg rotations possible. A spherical head from one bone fits into a circular socket from another to form a ball-and-socket joint. This is what allows for rotation and multi-directional movement.

Hinge Joints

Hinges joints allow for bending and straightening the body. They are found in the elbows and knees. For actions like running, walking, and lifting objects, they are necessary. Similar to a door hinge, these joints rotate on a single plane, providing the stability and strength required for walking and bearing weight.

Gliding Joints

In the wrists and the ankles, there gliding joints allow the bones to slide across one another in various directions. In the hands and feet, gliding joints provide the primary flexibility. These joints consist of flat or slightly curved parts of bones that rub against each other. This type of movement enhances the flexibility and maneuverability of these areas.

Pivot Joints

Rotation is possible at certain joints, including the one connecting the first and second cervical vertebrae. The head may be turned side to side thanks to pivot joints. With this kind of joint, rotation around a single axis is possible because the rounded end of one bone fits into a ring that is formed by another bone and surrounding ligament.

Condyloid Joints

These joints, which are located in the knuckles and wrists, allow for movement but not rotation. They permit the fingers and wrists to move in circles, bend, and straighten. Condyloid joints combine flexibility and stability by enabling flexion, extension, and a small amount of rotation of one bone's oval end into the hollow of another bone.

Saddle Joints

Saddle joints, which are found in the thumbs, allow for a grasping motion and enhance hand dexterity. They permit actions such as holding and gripping items. The concave and convex sections of saddle joints fit together like a rider in a saddle, allowing for movements in two planes—a critical feature for the intricate manipulations the thumb performs.

Bone Health and Disorders

Now, let us go deeper into the skeletal framework by examining some of the common bone diseases.

Throughout history, in order to understand human health issues, antiquarians and scientists have studied the composition of bones. Today, archeologists study skeleton remains so as to understand past communities, while biomedical researchers look at bone biology trying to find ways out for conditions such as osteoporosis or arthritis.

The bottom line is, in order to maintain overall wellness, one needs to have a healthy skeletal system. Proper nutrition, regular exercise, and avoiding injuries are critical elements for strong and effective bones that will help you live a longer and good quality life. Here are some of the most common diseases that impact the bone. Learning about them and how they come about will help you choose wiser approaches for enhancing your health and lifespan to the best of your ability.

Arthritis

More so a general term when used, arthritis means any condition that affects the joints. It has two major types which we've come to know as osteoarthritis and rheumatoid arthritis. Osteoarthritis typically takes some time to develop due to a progressive degenerative process which leads to the breakdown of the cartilage located on the ends of bones. This type is predominant in elderly persons and brings about general discomfort and restricted movements in the regions it affects. The synovium, the lining finish surrounding some human organs, especially the joints, is a form of auto-immune arthritis in in rheumatoid arthritis. This kind of arthritis tends to affect people of all ages. Its signs can include pain, joint inflammation, and, if left untreated, changes in the joint positions. In some extreme cases, one might need joint replacement or surgery to restore the joint, physical therapy to improve the continual use of the joint, or anti-inflammatory drugs.

Osteoporosis

Osteoporosis is a disease which is identified by thinning and brittle of bones, a condition in which bones break easily. This is disease common among people who are older because, as one's bone mass reduces, the body is unable to generate mass that is equal to the loss. Osteoporosis could also be caused by hereditary traits, low levels of calcium and vitamin D, too little or no exercise, smoking, and the overconsumption of alcohol. Osteoporosis primarily manifests itself in a higher likelihood of bone fractures in areas such as the hip, spine, or wrist. These fractures can cause a person to suffer from long-term pain, a reduction in stature, or event to bend forward with a curved back. Nutritional measures such as increased intake of calcium and vitamin D, weight bearing exercises, and alteration of lifestyle factors such as cessation of alcohol and smoking are perfect preventive measures.

Osteogenesis Imperfecta

Osteogenesis Imperfecta, commonly known as brittle bone disease, is a hereditary disorder where bones become easily frangible and fracture more often, sometimes with trivial or no provocation at all. It is due to genetic changes in the production of collagen, a protein well known to fashion strong bones. It is a severe illness and there is a big difference in the intensity among individuals. Some individuals may sustain just about five fractures in their lifetime, while others might sustain hundreds of them. Other features of the disease include blue-tinted sclera (the white part of the eye appears bluish), hearing loss, dental issues, and more frequent than normal fractures. Currently, there is no cure for the disease, making its treatment primarily focus on symptoms and fracture prevention. This might involve assistive devices for movement, physical therapy, or reconstruction involving bone grafts in extreme cases.

Paget's Disease

When a person is challenged with Paget's Disease, their bones get thicker, but paradoxically, they lose their strength and can be deformed. This disease usually occurs in individuals in their post-adolescence or elderly stage of life, and it is believed to be hereditary, though its origin is unknown. Paget's disease affects the regular remodeling process of bones, thus resulting in the generation of larger bone tissues. However, these bone tissues are weak and more vulnerable to fractures. Affected bones are most often the bones in the pelvis, skull, spine and legs. The signs and symptoms of skeletal involvement in leprosy are bone pain, joint pain, and deformities. In its complications, the continuous use of the jawbone can lead to arthritis, hearing impairment if the skull is involved, and increased incidence of bone cancer.

At this first stop, we have been able to cultivate a clear under-standing and explanation of the skeletal system and its formation, the various bones and joints present in the body, and the different diseases that befall our bones. You are now more informed to ensure that you do not remain idle and fail to take necessary actions that will help you maintain your bones. As we leave behind the sturdy framework of the skeletal system, get ready to head over to the next fascinating aspect of our body: the muscular system. We'll explore the mover behind our every action, from the smallest twitch to the heaviest lift. Buckle up! Our tour continues.

THE MUSCULAR SYSTEM

Here we are at the next destination of our tour through the human body. We are now at the muscular system. Consider your muscles like engines propelling a sleek, high-performance car; each muscle is carefully crafted to produce motion and power. Behind the scenes, our muscles work tirelessly, whether you are chopping up vegetables for dinner, jogging around the block, or simply smiling at friends. They are responsible for transforming energy into motion making everything we do possible.

At this stop we will be examining many different muscle groups and their specific roles. First, we'll get into the fact that are three types of muscles: skeletal, smooth, and cardiac muscles. We will also investigate how muscle fiber contraction works and how this marvel of nature's engineering makes movement possible. Lastly, this chapter also addresses common muscular conditions like strains and muscular dystrophy, highlighting ways to maintain healthy muscles.

Types of Muscles

Muscles are the movers and shakers of the body. They are tissues made of fibers that contract or relax based to produce movement in the body. Muscle tissues come in three distinct types that are located in just the right place to keep us moving. Here are the different muscle groups in your body:

Cardiac Muscles

These are the heart's diligent workers. Cardiac muscles work around the clock in your heart, not stopping for a moment, to pump blood through your body so that all cells get the oxygen and nourishment they need. Their longevity and their strength are evident in the way they beat from birth until death. What a muscle!

Skeletal Muscles

These are the muscles you see in action when you move. Attached to your bones by tendons, skeletal muscles control voluntary movements—actions you consciously control. So, whether you're lifting a box in your garage or running at the gym, these muscles are at work, showcasing their strength and flexibility.

Smooth Muscles

These are the introverts of the group, working quietly behind the scenes, but still making so much happen. Smooth muscles handle involuntary movements within your organs. Yes! Some of your organs move involuntarily. They help push food through your digestive tract, regulate blood flow by adjusting the diameter of your blood vessels, and even assist in the beauty of childbirth. Smooth muscles are indispensable for keeping our internal working and our body running "smoothly," just as the word suggests.

Muscle Anatomy and Function

Now, let's break down the topic of muscles further and zero in on how they help us move and stay active. Research articles on the topic wonderfully express:

> Your muscles are made of thousands of small fibers woven together. These fibers stretching and pressing together is what moves your organs or body. Your muscles weave together like a quilt that covers your body. They run in all directions and work together to move you. (Cleveland Clinic, 2021, para. 6)

So, let's get into the anatomy of the muscle. Or, in other words, what other body parts apart from the tissue come together to make the muscle.

Muscle Fibers

Muscles are like strings of super-tough fibers arranged in groups of numerous individual ropes. They can also be described as a type of flesh tissue that has the ability to contract as we touched on earlier. This tissue is immensely matted into smaller strands which are scientifically called myofibrils. These myofibrils are further split into subunits known as sarcomeres, that are the actual all-work-and-no-play in terms of muscles. When your muscles contract, the sarcomeres do all the work and guarantee that every movement is accurate and measured.

Tendons

Now on to tendons. These are the strong, cable-like bands which bind the muscles to the bones. They have the important role of converting force produced by a muscle contraction into movement. As your muscles contract, they drag these tendons, and thus the bones, which results in motion. This connection is necessary for any kind of motion; whether relative to the ground, like walking and jumping, or relative to objects, like holding and picking up a fork. Tendons are very strong structures and can handle a lot of tension and pressure to allow your body to keep functioning.

Connective Tissue

There is a layer called the endomysium that surrounds each individual muscle fiber. These aggregate into bundles ensheathed by another layer known as the perimysium, and then a layer above that called the epimysium. All these bundles are wrapped by the subsidiary epimysium, which appears to be a thicker layer of fat. It also encloses and safeguards the muscle fibers while transmitting the force generated by muscle contractions effectively. It is this protective strategy of having several layers of insulation wrapped around an electrical cable that ensures energy goes exactly where it's needed.

Sarcomeres

Finally, let us look at sarcomeres, the smallest part of muscle fibers responsible for muscle contraction. There are two major proteins that exist in sarcomeres called actin and myosin. You can just imagine these proteins as being the cogs in a large machine enabling it to run very smoothly. When your muscle receives a signal to contract, the actin and myosin slide along past one another in a shortening effect that generates force. It is a well-choreographed system that makes it possible for the body to move in a harmonious way.

Muscle Contractions

Now, let's discuss in greater detail how muscles function. Muscles contract and relax so that they can work properly; this function is under the nervous system's control through signals it sends to the muscles. When the decision is made to move a muscle, your brain will issue a signal over nerves that will cause muscle fibers to contract. This action is done by contraction and relaxation of the muscular fibers.

Types of Contractions

Isotonic Contraction: Muscles contract in order to alter their length and produce force. This includes:

- Concentric Contraction: Muscles get shorter as they pull their ends nearer together. An example is when lifting a weight.
- Eccentric Contraction: Muscles stretch with the contraction, such as when slowly letting go of a weight.

Isometric Contraction: Muscles generate force without changing their own length. This is experienced when holding a weight steady.

Energy for Contraction

Muscles need energy to work, which they gain through adenosine triphosphate (ATP). Even though some ATP is stored in muscles, most of it is produced by breaking down glucose and other nutrients as they are metabolized.

Muscle Growth and Repair

Exercise stimulates muscle hypertrophy, the enlargement of muscle fibers. Some stem cells known as satellite cells help to heal damaged muscles so as to boost healing or strengthen them.

Altogether, muscles are extraordinary for their capacity to transform energy into motion; they keep us active to accomplish different tasks throughout the day. Knowledge of the muscular system helps us to develop awareness of the workings of the human body.

Common Muscular Disorders

Strains and Sprains

Stretching of the muscles and ligaments can bring about one of the most common and prevalent disorders, sprains and strains. In the event that muscle fibers are overstretched, or even torn, one experiences a strain. The main causes of this are either overworking the muscle or some sort of abuse or neglect. Pain, edema, and stiffness in the afflicted muscles and surrounding tissues are signs of muscular strain. In some cases, seeking expert assistance is advised; for example, if there is significant swelling, if the symptoms do not improve with self-care, or if there is noticable derformity.

On the other hand, a sprain occurs to the ligament. These are tissues that connect the bones together in the joints. These are the groups of fibrous bands that, in a sprain, either become stretched or, as is often the case, actually ruptured due to a twist or some sort of blow. It is advisable to perform the first aid treatment method called the rest, ice, compression, and elevation (RICE) approach. This approach is best for soft tissue injuries like strains, sprains, and bruises. It involves resting the area to prevent further damage, applying ice to reduce the swelling and possibly numb the pain, compressing the area with a bandage to provide support, and elevating the injured area above the heart to reduce swelling. A person injured with a sprain or strain can also take pain-relieving medications and apply support or a brace to the affected part.

Fibromyalgia

Fibromyalgia is a chronic disorder that causes musculoskeletal pain, fatigue, and tenderness of the skin at different parts of the body. Much is still unknown, but, as before, it is assumed that this condition is caused by genes, along with environmental and psychological factors. Some of the signs include disturbed sleep patterns, disability to concentrate, and also increased tenderness.

Non-pharmacological treatment of fibromyalgia is comprised of the using pain relievers and sleep inducers, physiotherapy, workouts, and maintaining stress minimizing practices, among others. Cognitive behavioral therapy (CBT) is one of the many other treatments that can be of help when addressing this condition because of its characteristics of being chronic in nature.

Muscular Dystrophy

Muscular dystrophy is a general term for a number of inherited diseases whereby muscles progressively become weaker and then die. Notably, it is also significant to note that there are different types, but the most common one is Duchenne muscular dystrophy which usually affects males during early childhood. This condition arises from a deficiency in dystrophin (a protein that plays a key role in muscle function), due to genetic mutation. As a result, people with this deficiency ultimately develop walking, breathing, and other motor difficulties.

Muscular dystrophy is a chronic condition that is currently not curable, although patients can receive various therapies, medications, and equipment to alleviate some of the symptoms and lead more comfortable lives. In the meantime, advancements to treat this debilitating disorder and possibly a cure continue to be sought.

Tendinitis

Tendinitis, an inflammation of connective tissues that link muscles to bones, arises due to repetitive motions or sudden, severe injury. Symptoms include pain and swelling along the affected tendon that is often worse with motion. The most common regions for tendinitis comprise shoulders, elbows, wrists and knees.

The major aim in treating tendinitis is to minimize inflammation as well as reduce distress felt by a patient. It may involve rest, ice, anti-inflammatory medications, and physical therapy. In extreme situations, damaged tendons can be corrected through corticosteroid injections or even surgical operation.

Myasthenia Gravis

Myasthenia gravis is a muscular disorder resulting in fatigue and muscle weakness. Myasthenia gravis happens due to wrong response from immune system whereby it attacks nerve-muscle communications. Drooping eyelids, double vision, difficulty swallowing are some of the general symptoms of myasthenia gravis, which get worse from exercise but improve through relaxation.

Treatment for myasthenia gravis usually entails medicines that boost nerve-muscle communication, immunosuppressants to reduce immune system activity, and at times surgical removal of the thymus gland. Timely diagnosis and treatment are very important in managing symptoms effectively to improve one's quality of life.

As we come to the end of this stop, do not forget the importance of these muscles in the day-to-day functioning of your body. Each one of them is a behind-the-scenes superstar, unseen and unheard, yet vital for every event, minor or major. Are you ready to learn about the next major player in the human body?

THE NERVOUS SYSTEM

Here we are at the nervous system! Think, for a moment, of your brain and spinal cord as the headquarters of your central nervous system (CNS). Big decisions, such as whether to get up or snooze your alarm for the fifth time, are made there. The nervous system is a top-notch soldier that works tirelessly in the field, sending updates and messages from headquarters to the rest of the body.

> Every person's body contains billions of nerve cells (neurons). There are about 100 billion in the brain and 13.5 million in the spinal cord. The body's neurons take up and send out electric and chemical signals (electrochemical energy) to other neurons (Cirino, 2019, para. 3)

The chapter will ensure that you develop a deep appreciation for the intellectual processes of your mind, spine, and nerves. Let's plunge deep into this topic. Brace yourself for a mind-tickling adventure!

Central and Peripheral Nervous Systems

Imagine the CNS as the central hub in a city, a high-tech command center where critical decisions take place. This hub consists of the brain and spinal cord. The brain, our master controller, processes information, makes decisions, and coordinates actions.

It's like the CEO of your body, always in command, whether you're solving a complex math problem or deciding what to eat for dinner. It's that link without which no single signal could reach where it is supposed to go in a timely manner. The brain is the most efficient postal service ever known, moving important parcels of information.

Now let us go into the suburbs and countryside, where we find the peripheral nervous system (PNS). In comparison, the PNS works just like an army of people who have been positioned throughout a capital city to ensure all orders from their central offices are executed efficiently. It involves all nerves in the body, which stem from the spinal cord and brain and extend to every part of your body.

There are two divisions of PNS, namely somatic and autonomic systems. The somatic system controls voluntary movements such as typing, dancing, or giving someone a high five. It activates in order for you use your muscles, whenever you decide to. Meanwhile, the autonomic nervous system regulates involuntary activities such as the heartbeat, digestion, and the breathing process—those processes that happen on their own while we rarely notice them. It is like being behind the camera crew in a theater play; they make sure everything runs smoothly without the audience's knowledge.

Neurons and Synapses

Neurons are cells that are specialized in helping to transfer information within the body. Consider them as signal transmitting entities that convey core information with a high degree of speed and accuracy. They use electrical signals to transmit information.

When a neuron is activated and receives sufficient signals, there is a change in the electrical charge, which enables the neurons to communicate quickly. Let's learn about the three main parts of a neuron.

Cell Body (Soma)

This is the neuron's control center. It contains the nucleus and all its genetic material. Incoming signals are processed by the cell body, and this helps to maintain a healthy neuron.

Dendrites

These finger-like extensions receive information from other neurons. They act like tiny antennas to pick up messages and take them to the soma.

Axon

This thin, long thread carries signals away from the soma to other neurons, muscles, or glands. Axons may be short or very long, with some extending up to one meter in human beings. The ending of an axon has many terminal buttons that release neurotransmitters to pass on this electrical signal.

Synapses

The synapses are the small spaces in between neurons that are involved in transferring messages between neurons. It is commonly known as the synaptic connection or the gap between two neurons. After arriving at the end of the axon, a process takes place whereby specific chemicals known as neurotransmitters are released. They then diffuse across the synapse and bind to specific receptors located in dendrites of another neuron, thus ensuring that the transfer of signals is continuous. There are two main types of synapses:

Chemical Synapses

These are the most common synapse. When an electrical impulse gets to the terminal button (the small bulb at the end of an axon), it brings about the release of neurotransmitters over the synaptic cleft (a space between two neurons).

Electrical Synapses

This synapse is rarer. When it happens, neurons are connected through mechanisms known as gap junctions that allow easy transmission of electric impulses between neurons. This kind of synapse permits very fast signal transfer as compared to the chemical synapses.

Neurological Disorders

Neurological diseases impact the proper functioning of the brain. It is important to be aware of these disorders in order to recognize them and treat them. Anyone can have a neurological disorder, but they can differ greatly in degree of severity and affect different areas of life for different patients. Here is a brief overview of some of the more well-known neurological disorders, what they are, and how one might go about getting treatment for them and even engage in prevention.

Alzheimer's Disease

Alzheimer's is a disease that you might know something about. This is an umbrella term that refers to a class of dementia in which clinical manifestation includes the worsening of one's memories, thinking abilities, behavior, and interactions with others. Describing the experience in an article titled "Life with Dementia: My Family's Experience," Warren Alexander-Pye shared:

> Caring for someone at home is difficult and exhausting. The forgetfulness is initially a bit 'quirky' but develops into something which becomes a lot more emotionally entangled. Things which have been misplaced moved from 'lost' to 'stolen' and accusations were made which were hurtful when you were only trying to help. The person with dementia feels in some way violated but can't describe either reason or cause. People and places from forty, fifty and sixty years ago become real and present again whilst the events of yesterday are forgotten. You are no longer recognized as a family member and any sense of gratitude is lost. (Alexander-Pye, 2016, para. 4)

The root cause of this disease is not known, but it is agreed that there are genetic, environmental, as well as lifestyle predisposing factors to the disease. Age is the main risk factor, as the probability of getting the disease rises sharply at the age of 65 and above. Other factors associated with the disease are a history of injuries in the head or previous traumas, unhealthy diet, physical inactivity, and tobacco use.

Alzheimer's is progressive, and the symptoms can become relatively severe. The first symptoms are short-term memory problems, perplexity, problems with familiar activities, and difficulties with speaking. In its advanced stage, such patients suffer from severe memory loss other behavioral changes. These patients may not even recognize their relatives and friends; they may not be able to perform simple tasks on their own.

Alzheimer's, unfortunately, cannot be cured at the moment, though there are medications and therapies for controlling the manifestations of the disease. Other drugs such as cholinesterase inhibitors and memantine are useful in treating memory loss and other related problems. Creating a safe environment, engaging in certain cognitive-training activities, and using tools daily to assist in improving memory are also helpful options.

Epilepsy

Epilepsy is a neurological disorder that involves episodes and attacks that are sudden and unprovoked. A seizure, to zero in on the condition, is a transient event that involves the brain and manifests in different ways in terms of movement, emotion, and level of awareness.

Common factors contributing to epilepsy are genetic factors, cerebral trauma, other diseases including cancer and strokes, viral encephalitis, birth injuries, and developmental disorders such as autism. Risk factors include age (more common in young children and older adults), family history, head injuries, stroke and other vascular diseases, brain infections, and prolonged seizures in childhood.

Seizure symptoms can vary widely from temporary confusion to staring spells with irresistible jerking movements of the arms and legs to loss of consciousness/awareness, and psychic symptoms (such as fear, anxiety, and déjà vu). Seizures can occur anywhere within the brain, therefore, how they manifest differs depending on which region is affected.

Epilepsy treatment often includes medications for preventing seizures through anti-seizure drugs prescribed to decrease the frequency and intensity. Surgical procedures, such as removing the part of the brain causing the seizure or the implantation of a vagus nerve stimulation device, have also proven effective for some individuals. Other adjustments include getting ample sleep, managing stress, and avoiding potential triggers where possible. If recommended, dietary treatments like the ketogenic diet may help manage seizures.

Migraines

Most of us have experienced a migraine at least once in our lives. Am I right? That never-ending, pulsating pain in the head, often accompanied by feeling sick, vomiting, and a heightened sensitivity to bright light or loud sounds.

What causes migraines is not known for sure, but it is believed that they are influenced by genetic factors. Changing in the brainstem functioning and its interactions with the trigeminal nerve might also be involved in the origin of the disease. Triggers such as hormonal changes during menstruation periods, foods and drinks (for example aged cheese, alcohol, or red wine particularly), stress, sensory stimuli, such as strong odors from perfume, can provoke such an attack. Family history of migraines, age (usually between 30 and 40 years old), sex (women are more likely to get migraines), and hormonal fluctuations are some of the common risk factors.

The typical stages that migraines occur in are aura, where there are visual disturbances such as flashing lights flash or a zigzag pattern; blinding headaches that sometimes cause nausea and are painful when exposed to light, or loud noise, and postdrome—the "migraine hangover" that results in fatigue or confusion even once the migraine itself has stopped.

Treatment for migraines entails both symptomatic relief as well as prevention. Off-the-counter pain relievers, for instance ibuprofen and aspirin, could be used for acute symptoms, while prescription drugs like triptans are more effective alternatives. On the preventative end, some persons rely on beta-blockers, antidepressants, or anti-seizure drugs that help to decrease the frequency and severity of attacks. It is also useful to avoid the triggers that you know affect you, such as fatigue due to lack of sleep or skipping meals, high caffeine intake, especially through sodas, dehydration, and stress.

Multiple Sclerosis (MS)

MS is an autoimmune disease affecting the CNS, more particularly the brain and the spinal cord. With MS, the myelin sheath that surrounds nerves is damaged by the body's own immune system. This results in disconnection of signal exchange between different body parts and the brain, which may lead to permanent nerve damage or loss.

While researchers do not yet fully understand what causes this disease, it is thought to be an autoimmune disorder in which the body's immune system acts against normal tissue. It has been hypothesized by some scientists that such processes might be set off by environmental agents such as viral infections and one's genes.

Some of the other causes that have been identified include genetics, some diseases, age (the majority of patients acquire MS during their intermediate years), gender (women are more likely to get MS than men), and low levels of vitamin D.

The manifestations of MS can be easily explained; nevertheless, they depend on which nerves are involved and the amount of demyelinated axons. They include trembling of the arms and legs, difficulty walking, dizziness, fatigue, numbness or weakness in one or more limbs, loss of part or whole vision, painful eye movements, persistent abnormal double vision, tingling or pain in specific areas, and electric shock-like sensations when the neck is flexed.

There is no cure for MS, but its progression can be influenced through treatment aimed at managing symptoms. Nerve inflammations can be reduced by using drugs like corticosteroids, while relapses can be made less severe with the help of disease modifying therapies (DMTs). Physiotherapy treatments, along with muscle relaxants, can aid in relieving stiffness and spasticity in the muscles. Additionally, lifestyle adjustments such as regularly exercising, eating balanced diets, and learning how to manage stress have been proven helpful, too.

Parkinson's Disease

Parkinson's disease is a chronic neurological illness that mainly impacts communication between nerve cells and the brain. It progresses slowly, in some cases, with the initial symptom being trembling in one's hand that is almost unnoticeable. Though it is characterized by the occurrence of tremors, the disorder also has a tendency of resulting in rigidity or slowness of movement.

This occurs because the neurons in a specific area of the brain, known as the substantia nigra, are lost, which reduces the body's levels of dopamine. The list of causes leading to this type of degeneration is not fully understood and could be a result of genetic mutations, the environment in which the patient lives, and Lewy bodies, which are small protein formations inside brain cells. Some other causes are age (most people fall ill at the age of 60 or above), heredity, sex (it is more common in men than in women), and prolonged exposure to toxins such as pesticides and herbicides.

The common presentation of Parkinson's disease includes tremors, bradykinesia (slow movement), rigidity, postural instability, a masked or expressionless face, speech and writing abnormalities, hypophonia (abnormally weak vocal quality), and micrographia (impaired motor activity). Symptoms develop over time and, as the ailment progresses, the performance of daily tasks is affected.

Currently, Parkinson's disease cannot be cured, but the patient is often given drugs that help to alleviate the manifestations of the illness. These include increasing dopamine levels or mimicking its effects. Undergoing deep brain stimulation (DBS), which is the implantation of electrodes to the part of the brain that regulates movements in advanced Parkinson's patients, is also an option. Physical therapy, occupational therapy, and lifestyle changes, such as exercising and consuming healthy food, can also be safe treatments.

Is it safe to say that we now have a fair understanding of the nervous system? If so, then it's time for us to now learn about the circulatory system. This next stop is all about your heart, blood vessels, and all other players involved in keeping blood moving freely about your body.

THE CIRCULATORY SYSTEM

Among the undeniable facts, the circulatory system is one of the most complicated systems of the body. This core system functions by constantly circulating blood throughout the body. The blood also acts as the transport medium for substances like the oxygen and carbon dioxide, which are vital to our bodies' cells. The circulatory system is comprised of blood vessels, blood, and the heart as one of the main components. In order for circulation to take place efficiently, the key parts work together with other organs of the body to distribute oxygen and nutrients while removing harmful waste substances.

Heart Anatomy and Function

The heart is an extremely powerful muscle located in the chest region, slightly towards the left side from the middle. About the size of one's fist, it may not seem very powerful, but there is much to its work. It uses mainly two circuits, the systemic circulation and pulmonary circulation, to perform its main function of pumping blood. Pumping oxygenated blood into every organ occurs in systemic circulation, whereas deoxygenated blood is collected from all over through pulmonary circulation before the lungs expel carbon dioxide.

Chambers of the Heart

The heart is also divided into four chambers: the right atrium and right ventricle on the right side and the left atrium and left ventricle on the left. The atria is also found in the upper chambers of the heart while the ventricles are located in the lower chambers. The atria presents itself like the front porch of the heart, or like two-front doors through which blood arriving from its circulation journey is let in. The right atrium is always on standby to receive oxygen-depleted blood from the inferior and superior vena cava (one of two large veins that carry deoxygenated blood from the body back to the heart), while the left atrium accepts the oxygenated blood from the pulmonary veins (blood vessels that carry oxygenated blood from the lungs to the heart).

Blood Flow Through the Heart

Deeper in the heart there are the two ventricles we touched on earlier. They function as strong pumping chambers. The right ventricle does its part amazingly by pumping oxygen-low blood to the lungs through the pulmonary artery. In the lungs, this blood gains oxygen. It also trades off by shedding carbon dioxide. The left ventricle, the most muscular and strongest wall of the heart, pumps the oxygenated blood through aorta, which is the largest artery. The left wall is much thicker to exert the pressure that is necessary to pump blood all over the body.

Blood Vessels and Circulation

Blood, which we know delivers substances to cells and removes cell waste, is a fluid specialized in transporting. It is not only the red liquid which comes from us when we injure ourselves; it includes red blood cells, white blood cells, platelets and plasma. It transports oxygen throughout the body, since it is full of hemoglobin, which is formed with oxygen in the lungs. On the other hand, white blood cells are among the immune cells in the body, assisting in fighting infections and other diseases. Platelets are involved in clotting, which prevents excessive bleeding when a person is injured, and plasma is a liquid component that carries cells, among other substances, such as nutrients hormones, and waste products.

Meanwhile, blood vessels are the modus operandi transportation terminal in the circulatory system, comprised of the arteries, veins, and capillaries. All three have their own jobs, which are all very important. Arteries are blood vessels with thick walls that transport oxygenated blood from the heart (which is like the terminal's center) to other organs of the body. They must be tough like durable rubber hoses and stretchy enough like elastic bands to deal with the high levels of pressure that occur when the heart pumps blood through them. In contrast, veins carry non-oxygenated blood back to the heart. They have less thickness than arteries and usually possess valves that check reverse flow so that the correct passage of blood is ensured. Capillaries are minute, thin-walled tubes where gases, nutrition, and waste products are exchanged. These link arterial parts to venous parts, hence allowing oxygen with nutrients into tissues, while dealing with waste management.

Despite all of this amazing teamwork from the blood vessels, the heart requires some system that allows it to direct blood flow, causing it to move in a single direction. This is where valves come in. They allow blood to pass through the heart but not flow backwards, which is a very important job in the grander scheme of things. Their four primary valves can be found in the circulatory system, and they are the the aortic valve, tricuspid valve, pulmonary valve, and the mitral valve.

- Tricuspid Valve: The tricuspid valve can be found snug between the right atrium and right ventricle. It goes into action and seals off its passage way to stop the back flow of blood into the atrium whenever the ventricular contracts.
- Pulmonary Valve: The pulmonary valve, on the other hand, can be found between the right ventricle and the pulmonary artery. It allows some amount of blood to pass to the lungs, but then it firmly shuts, similarly preventing any back flow.
- Mitral Valve: Found on the left between left atrium and left ventricle, the mitral is like a double action door. It serves as a gateway for blood entering or leaving ventricles, preventing a reverse flow.
- Aortic Valve: Lastly, the aorta connects with left ventricle by means of aortic valve, which permits oxygenated blood to spread round the body when it opens and prevents the blood from returning back to heart during closure.

Apart from these valves, the superior and inferior vena cava are two principal veins that perform the function of bringing back oxygenated blood in all parts of our bodies. They flow into the right atrium. From there, blood that lacks oxygen goes back to the heart through the superior and inferior vena cava and is taken to the right atrium. In a nutshell, all other parts of the body get oxygen from aorta, which discharges pure blood coming from the left ventricle, whereas waste products generated by these two ventricles are carried off by arteries carrying deoxygenated blood.

Blood and Its Components

Blood might make some of us feel uneasy, often bringing thoughts of pain or injury to mind. But there's a pretty interesting story beyond what meets the eye. Blood is like a delivery service. Your very own DoorDash, UPS, or FedEx that ensures every part of our body gets the nutrients it placed an order for. This is all thanks an amazing team of dedicated workers who work around the clock, no days off: your red blood cells, white blood cells, platelets, and plasma. We've mentioned these before, but how about we learn, in detail, what each one does?

Red Blood Cells (RBCs/ Erythrocytes)

The red blood cell, which is also called an erythrocyte, is the predominant type of cell in the blood. It constitutes about 40-45% of its volume. These cells are transporters because they move carbon dioxide to the lungs where it is exhaled, and oxygen from lungs to other parts of the body. With the red blood cell's two concave faces, it has a large surface area for conducting this gaseous exchange.

In red blood cells there is a substance known as haemoglobin, which combines with oxygen in the lungs by releasing where it is most needed. Haemoglobin carries carbon dioxide back to the lungs, a waste product during metabolism. It has been found that, after approximately 120 days, red blood cells disintegrate, either in the liver or spleen, and those parts break down to form new cells.

White Blood Cells (WBCs/ Leukocytes)

Leukocytes or white blood cells mainly work to offer basic protection against diseases in the body. They are important players within the immune system. Despite being only one percent prevalent within the blood, their effects are tangible. There are various types of white blood cells, each having specific roles:

Neutrophils

These are the most abundant among WBCs, accounting for 50-70%ot. They are most active during the early stages of an infection, where processes such as phagocytosis (engulfing of solid particles) occur to eliminate bacteria.

Lymphocytes

These occur in the course of adaptive immunity. There are B cells, which secrete antibodies that neutralize pathogens, and are dangerous to bacteria and viruses. On the other hand, there are T cells, which destroy the cancerous or infected cells.

Monocytes

On leaving the bloodstream, monocytes turn into macrophages (immune cells that engulf and digest pathogens and cellular debris) as well as dendritic cells, which are found in various organs. In other words, they contribute much in terms of phagocytosis and hold the antigens in place to help with immune system coordination.

Eosinophil

These cells are major fighters against parasites and also play a role in allergic reactions.

Basophil

These are the least abundant WBCs and produce histamine (a chemical causing inflammation) during allergic reactions that causes an inflammatory response that leads to swelling.

Platelets (Thrombocytes)

Platelets called thrombocytes are responsible for blood clotting and are small disc-shaped cell fragments. Platelets form part of a chain reaction initiated by injury to a vessel; they arrive first like real-life paramedics or first aid workers. They congregate at the damaged area, then aggregate and deliver molecular signals that trigger the coagulation cascade process.

Coagulation cascade is basically a group of reactions that cause the formation of a clot in blood that helps to stop bleeding on the site of the vessels that were affected. Platelets also secrete growth factors that assist in remodeling and new tissue formation in areas that contain injuries. Platelets are relatively small than RBCs, and they live for only about 7-10 days; the function of platelets is very essential in the maintenance of the integrity of the circulatory system.

Plasma

This free-flowing liquid material consists of about 55% of the total volume of blood; it is called plasma. It is a pale yellow fluid originating from the liver which acts as a vehicle for transporting nutrients, hormones, and waste products in the body. Water and other contents constituting plasma are approximately 92% and 8% respectively. These contents include proteins, electrolytes, gases, nutrients and wastes.

Key components of plasma include:

Albumin

Albumin is a main plasma protein that helps maintain osmotic pressure, which is crucial for keeping fluid within blood vessels. At the same time, it transports different hormones and drugs, among other substances, through circulation.

Globulins

This type of protein consists of antibodies, commonly referred to as immunoglobulins, that play a crucial role in immune response mechanisms. Some of the other globulins carry lipids, hormones, and other molecules with them.

Fibrinogen

Fibrinogen is an important clotting factor that, through the coagulation process, gets converted into fibrin, which gives the blood clot its structural feature.

Electrolytes

Plasma is composed of water, salts, proteins, vitamins, and various, other substances, including sodium, potassium, calcium, bicarbonate, chloride ions, and many others, which are electrolytes. For optimum functioning, these ions regulate pH levels, nerve impulses, and muscle contractions.

Nutrients and Waste Products

Plasma also helps in carrying nutrients from the digestive system, such as glucose, amino acids, and vitamins, to all the cells in the body. It also transports waste products such as urea and creatinine to the kidneys for excretion.

Hormones

Plasma also acts as a transport medium for hormones produced by endocrine glands to help in conveying signals between various organs.

CARDIOVASCULAR DISORDERS

A large number of diseases that affect the heart and blood vessels fall under cardiovascular disorders, which are very risky to health and affect many individuals worldwide. Prevention and control require an in-depth comprehension of these conditions, their causes, symptoms, as well as treatments.

Heart Failure

Also referred to as congestive heart failure, this occurs when the heart fails to pump blood effectively, causing inadequate circulation to meet the body's requirements. This may be due conditions that weaken or overwork the heart like coronary heart disease (CAD), hypertension, or previous myocardial infarction (heart attack). Symptoms may include shortness of breath, fatigue, swollen legs or feet, and rapid or irregular heartbeats. To treat this condition, it mainly involves changing one's lifestyle, medication for reducing symptoms and improving cardiac function, and possibly the surgical insertion of devices like pacemakers or implantable cardioverter-defibrillators (ICDs).

Arrhythmias

Electrical malfunctions within your heart cause arrhythmias, which are irregular beating patterns often noticed when you have a series of faulty pulses transmitted by your EKG machine. These irregular beating patterns could range from harmless to life-threatening and include conditions such as atrial fibrillation, bradycardia, and ventricular tachycardia (VT). You may get these from various factors, which include CAD, electrolyte imbalances related to some drugs, and congestive heart failure (CHF), among others. Palpitations could be experienced, where small electric shocks run through your chest wall, while you might also become dizzy after exhaling heavily. Treatment involves the use of drugs, changes in lifestyle, electrical cardioversion for the conversion of the heart rhythm to normal, or even surgical interventions, such as ablation to correct the heart's timing.

Hypertension (High Blood Pressure)

High blood pressure, or hypertension as it is commonly referred to, is one of the world's leading cardiovascular diseases. It is characterized by the continually high force of blood against the arterial walls. If left uncontrolled, it causes life-threatening diseases such as heart disease, stroke, and kidney failure. The problem tends to gradually develop over time without any presentation until later stages. Hypertensive risk factors include obesity, lack of physical activity, alcoholism, consuming too much salt, and family history. But some signs can be unseen, though others may be visible. For example, constant headaches, breathlessness, sneezing and nose bleeding. Treatment for high BP involves changing one's diet, engaging in regular exercises, reducing salt consumption, and using prescribed medications for lowering high blood pressure.

Congenital Heart Defects (CHD)

Structural abnormalities in the heart from birth are referred to as congenital heart defects. These could be simple like small openings in the heart wall or complex such as absence of parts or malformation of tissues making up the organ itself. The origin of CHD remains largely unknown, though genetic factors play a role, together with environmental exposure leading to gene mutation. Symptoms will vary depending on the kind and severity but can include blue skin coloration known as cyanosis, rapid breathing rates, fatigue, and more, such as poor growth observed in children suffering from congenital heart disease. This is among the possible reasons why there seems to be growth challenges seen among children and adolescents with CAD when compared against their peers without any major physiological illnesses. Treatment options range from monitoring only or using medicines to surgical interventions aimed at correcting these deformities.

Heart Valve Disease

When one or more valves do not work properly, thus affecting blood flow within the heart, this condition is known as heart valve disease. For instance, valve stenosis (narrowing) and valve regurgitation (leakage). These can be caused by defects at birth, rheumatic fever, infective endocarditis, and changes linked with age progression. The signs vary but commonly include tiredness, breathlessness, swollen ankles/feet, and sometimes chest pains. Management options depend on how severe the symptoms are. Medications might be given just to control symptoms while surgical procedures such as repairing/replacing damaged valves could also become necessary.

Coronary Artery Disease

Coronary artery disease, also known as ischemic heart disease, is caused by plaque build-up in the coronary arteries that feed the heart with blood. The narrowing of these arteries reduces the flow of blood to the heart resulting in chest pain (angina), breathlessness, and heart attack. It can be caused by high cholesterol levels, hypertension, smoking, diabetes, and physical inactivity. CAD treatment usually involves lifestyle changes, medications for symptom control, and reduction of atherosclerosis and sometimes surgical procedures such as angioplasty or coronary artery bypass graft (CABG) surgery to restore normal blood flow.

Stroke

When the supply of blood to a section of the brain is blocked or reduced, it results in a stroke. This can be due to an artery that has been obstructed (ischaemic stoke) or a blood vessel that has developed leaks or bursts (haemorrhagic stroke). Hypertension, smoking, diabetes mellitus, hyperlipidemia, as well as atrial fibrillation may trigger the disorder. Stroke symptoms include abrupt numbness or weakness, especially on one side of the body, confusion, difficulty speaking or understanding speech, and loss of balance or coordination. Immediate medical attention is necessary for reducing brain damage and enhancing outcomes. Long-term care might entail drugs, lifestyle modifications, and rehabilitation therapies to restore lost capacities.

Healthier lifestyle choices, like staying active or being cautious about your diet, are some of the things that can help us to keep this vital system running smoothly on a daily basis. Now, it's time for us to move forward on our tour and check out the respiratory system. Like blood keeps moving thanks to the circulatory system, the respiratory system ensures that blood is oxygenated and ready to fuel every motion we make.

THE RESPIRATORY SYSTEM

Guess what? We're now at the mid-point of our one-of-a-kind tour of the human body. We'll now be learning about the respiratory system. Think of your most recent breath. In that short moment, an amazing process happened whereby life-giving air was sucked into your lungs and carbon dioxide was removed from them. The respiratory system is an amazing design of biology and plays a key role in preserving life by balancing gases.

Our lungs are located in the chest cavity. They are two spongy organs which are the central players within this system; protected by the ribcage, they help us breathe all day long. Air enters either via the nostrils or mouth before descending along the windpipe, dividing at bronchi, then finally reaching tiny sacs called alveoli. This is where carbon dioxide gets exchanged with oxygen during inhalation.

The respiratory system, however, goes beyond just being a series of air passages and organs. It helps us to speak by passing air through vocal cords in the larynx, which produce sounds and enable communication. Additionally, the respiratory system warms, filters, and humidifies incoming air that protects lungs from harmful particles as well as pathogens. Moreover, it also acts as an acid-base regulator by controlling carbon dioxide levels within blood and even plays some part in olfactory sense, since air passes through the nasal passageways, thereby stimulating olfactory receptors.

I can't wait for us to go deeper into this amazing system!

Structure of the Respiratory System

As all the systems that we have learned about, the respiratory system is also divided into several parts all having their roles. They all require each other for optimal performance of the entire system. For the respiratory system, there are six main parts that we'll come to understand.

Nose

At the start of our journey is the nose, which is how air gets into our body. The nose has three main roles: filtering, warming, and moistening inhaled air. The external part of the nose, as seen on our faces, is made of bone and cartilage leading to the nostril openings. Right inside the nostrils are fine hairs (cilia) that keep any large particles like dirt and other debris from entering the respiratory tract.

Air then passes through the nasal cavity, a big hollow space at the back of the nose. This cavity contains mucus membranes that excrete mucus to prevent dust, germs, and other small particles from going further in. Furthermore, there are many blood vessels within this section that warm up air to body temperature before it enters deep into the lungs. Also found here are olfactory cells that provide a sense of smell.

Pharynx

Later on, air moves down into the pharynx, which links both respiratory and digestive systems by means of a muscular tube. There are three parts of the pharynx: nasopharynx (upper area at rear end inside nasal), oropharynx (middle part at behind mouth), and laryngopharynx (inferior region leading to the larynx and esophagus).

The nasopharynx allows air to move through the nasal cavity to the next section of the pharynx. It houses adenoids that trap pathogens that cause infections. The oropharynx serves two functions. Food passes through the oropharynx while going towards the stomach, though it can also be used for breathing purposes, as well. The last section, called the laryngopharynx, helps guide food to the esophagus, which will eventually lead to digestion. It also allows air to pass through the larynx.

Larynx

The larynx, which is also referred to as the voice box, is the spot where air finally arrives. This organ is found at the far end of the trachea, and it has various roles like sound production, protecting airways, and guiding air into the trachea. The larynx consists of numerous cartilages, along with the Adam's apple, which is a common name for the thyroid cartilage.

Located in this part of the respiratory system are vocal cords. These stretch across the passage through which air flows. When we breathe out through our vocal cords, they vibrate, causing sounds. The tension and length of our vocal cords determine how high or low our pitch will be, while their thicknesses typically control our voices' loudness. Inside, there's also a door that seals off the windpipe when we swallow anything.

Trachea

Afterwards, air goes down to the trachea, known as windpipe. The trachea has C-shaped pieces of cartilage that are positioned around its walls, allowing it to keep its shape and remain open all the time. Along its interior surface are also ciliated cells and mucus-producing goblet cells responsible for trapping foreign materials similar to those found in nasal cavities.

The trachea serves as a connecting link between the larynx and bronchi, providing passage ways for air transportation from one region to another. Similarly, it aids in keeping diseases from affecting the lower respiratory system. The cilia move trapped particles upwards towards the pharynx where they can be swallowed or coughed up.

Bronchi

Afterwards, the trachea splits into two bronchi: the left and right bronchi, which lead to the lungs. Bronchi are also supported by cartilage rings and lined with cilia and mucus to maintain the filtering of air. Going further inside, on one side of the lung, there is a primary bronchus which subdivides into secondary bronchi leading to each lobe of the lung (three on the right; two on the left). They, in turn, subdivide into even smaller bronchi tertiary that we call bronchioles.

Bronchioles have smooth muscles in their walls and lack cartilage, relying on these muscles to hold their structure. These minute tubes continue to branch in an intricate pattern ensuring air will reach every part of the lungs.

Lungs

As we briefly discussed, these organs are located in your body on the two sides of your chest. Lungs are spongy, having an elastic feature that allows them to expand and contract with each breath taken. A double-layered membrane called pleura serves as a protective covering around the lungs. The pleura secretes a fluid that helps moisten the space between its layers, which minimizes friction during breathing.

Inside it, the bronchiole ends by dividing into tiny air sacs called alveoli clusters, present in the millions in each lung. There are about 300 million alveoli within each lung. The alveolar walls are a combination of capillaries. Oxygen in the air entering the lungs is able to pass through the alveolar wall to get to the blood, while carbon passes through the alveolar walls to get out as air being exhaled.

While we can live without a lung, a nose, and even a larynx, these are all very important parts of the respiratory system that make life easier. Now, zeroing in on what the respiratory system is most known for, we'll learn about the mechanics of breathing.

Mechanics of Breathing

Respiration is a process in which breathing occurs because several muscles, structures, and pressures work together. This process can be broadly divided into two main phases: inspiration and expiration. It will be interesting to go through each of these phases to discover the exquisite processes that occur when we breathe.

Inhalation (Inspiration)

Inhalation can be defined as the manner by which human respires or how we draw air into the lungs.

Diaphragm

Size wise, the diaphragm is the largest muscle of the body. It is dome shaped, extending from the thoracic or chest cavity to the abdominal cavity. This muscle is regarded as the most significant one due to the actions that are performed during breathing. During inhalation, the diaphragm lowers itself to expand space inside thoracic cavity. This contraction originates from the phrenic nerve, which starts at neck level before proceeding downwards towards the diaphragm.

External Intercostal Muscles

These groups of muscles lie between ribs. During their contraction they raise the ribcage upwards and outwards, thus further increasing volume within thoracic cavity. This action also enhances the lung's expansion.

According to Pulmonary Associates, most people don't know that when their chest moves up and down it's not directly because air is entering the lung.

> Chest movement during breathing isn't the result of air movement. When you breathe in, our chest swells; when you breathe out, our chest collapses. But these chest movements are not actually the result of air filling up or exiting the lungs. During inhalation, the diaphragm—a thin sheet of dome-shaped muscle that separates the chest and abdominal cavities—contracts and moves down, increasing the space in the chest cavity. At the same time, the muscles between the ribs contract to pull the rib cage upward and outward. During exhalation, the exact opposite happens (Pulmonary Associates, 2017).

When the thoracic cavity volume decreases, there is an increase in the pressure inside the lungs (intrapulmonary pressure). This rise in pressure causes air to be pushed out of the lungs by following Boyle's Law, which states that the pressure of a gas is inversely proportional to its volume. The air then reverses its path: from the alveoli, through the bronchioles and bronchi, up the trachea, and out through the nose or mouth.

However, there are other muscles that come into play when forced exhalation occurs. Passive expiry is done during quiet breathing, while forced expiration, which could be like blowing candles or participating in any vigorous exercise, can require additional muscles activity.

Gas Exchange in the Alveoli

Gas exchange is among the most fundamental roles of the respiratory system, occurring within small air sacs called alveoli found in the lungs. This process supplies oxygen to the blood and gets rid of carbon dioxide, which are necessary for sustaining life.

Structure of Alveoli

Alveoli are microscopic sacs found at the tips of bronchioles, surrounded by dense capillary network. Each lung contains about 300 million alveolar sacs, allowing for a huge surface area for gaseous diffusion. The wall of these structures is extremely thin, made up only of one layer epithelial cells (cells that line various surfaces of the body) allowing easy passage for gases through them.

Process of Gas Exchange

- Inhalation: Air enters into our bodies as we breathe in through respiratory tract until it reaches alveolus where oxygen concentration is higher than that present around capillaries, creating concentration gradient.
- Oxygen Diffusion: Oxygen molecules move through the walls separating alveolar spaces from neighboring capillaries so that they can get into contact with the haemoglobin contained inside red blood cells. After binding together with RBCs, the oxyhemoglobin now formed is carried all over the body where it is needed for respiration.
- Carbon Dioxide Removal: At the same time, carbon dioxide, a metabolic waste, is found in relatively rich

quantities in the blood coming to the lungs as compared to that in the air in alveoli. This concentration gradient means that carbon dioxide diffuses out of the capillaries into the alveoli.

- Exhalation: When a person breathes out the air that is rich in CO_2, that air goes along the bronchi and trachea, then out of the body.

Role of Hemoglobin

Transportation of gases within the body relies on red blood cells containing haemoglobin, which act as a carrier molecule for both oxygen as well carbon dioxide. Each molecule can combine with four molecules of oxygen, thus increasing its capacity to bind oxygen greatly and raising the levels available in circulation. Simultaneously, it picks carbon dioxide from tissues where it will then be taken towards the lungs so that it may get exhaled.

Factors Affecting Breathing Efficiency

Breathing can be affected by the position, activities that one is undergoing, and even conditions within the environment in which one is located. It is important to know these aspects and the measures that could be taken to promote effective breathing.

Posture

Different body postures have definitive effects on lung capacity and the breathing process. Sitting or standing curved or bending forward are among the most common postures that restrict chest expansion, making it difficult to take deeper breaths. Bad posture implies restriction of the chest cage and the capacity to breathe freely and deeply.

Physical Activity

Physical exercise is known to strengthen muscles of the respiratory system, such as the diaphragm and other intercostal muscles, making them more efficient. During exercise, the need for oxygen increases, hence the increased rate and depth of breathing.

Environmental Conditions

The quality of the air that is within our environment equally determines our rate of respiratory efficiency. Bacteria, viruses, dust and other particles in the air can cause irritation or swelling and constriction of the bronchi, hampering one's breathing. Other conditions, such as high-altitude pressure accompanied with low oxygen demand or availability can cause the respiratory system to pump harder in order to oxygenate the blood.

Diseases and Disorders

Different pulmonary conditions and illnesses affect the technique of breathing, thus decreasing its effectiveness and the amount of oxygen exchange. Asthma, COPD, and other respiratory illnesses can create inflammation, narrowing the airway due to mass formation.

Respiratory Health and Disorders

The overall wellness of the body depends on maintaining a healthy respiratory system because our lungs supply oxygen to all parts of the body and remove carbon dioxide. Various factors can affect respiratory health; they may be from personal choices or surroundings that one is exposed to.

Furthermore, common ailments also exist that can lead to serious health problems by limiting lung functions. We will therefore discuss how we can stay healthy with our breathing and look at some disorders that could interfere with this vital organ.

Respiratory Health Maintenance

There are some habits you can adopt which will help keep your lungs in good condition as well as prevent any possible diseases from attacking them so frequently:

Quit Smoking

Among many hazards associated with smoking is chronic obstructive pulmonary disease (COPD) caused by inhaling chemicals found in cigarette smoke over time, such as tar or nicotine among others. This condition often leads to developing lung cancer among other fatal illnesses. It's therefore important not only to quit smoking but to also try avoiding being near people who smoke, since secondhand smoke poses equal risks against respiratory wellness.

Regular Exercise

For all systems to work properly, including the breathing process, physical activity should always be part of your life. Examples of regular exercises that can be practiced are walking, jogging, swimming, and cycling, which strengthen the muscles around the chest, allowing you to take in more air when you inhale. At the same time, enhancing oxygen utilization efficiency within cells through increased breathing rate from general workout sessions is also very effective. Another fact is that exercise contributes to cardiovascular development, which directly impacts the proper working capacity of various organs, especially those involved in breathing, such as the heart and blood vessels.

Healthy Eating Habits

A balanced diet consisting mainly of fruits, vegetables grains, meats, and more, providing the necessary nutrients required for healthy lungs. Additionally, these food types contain antioxidants, known to reduce inflammation levels and safeguard against damage. Staying hydrated also ensures the mucus lining passages remain moist, making it easy for phlegm to move out through coughing or sneezing and preventing congestion build up that can result into infections.

Personal Cleanliness

It's advisable to always wash hands with soap under running water as often as possible, especially after visiting toilets, before eating meals, and whenever one comes into contact with unclean surfaces such as floors or dirty objects. Failure to do so may lead to the direct transfer of germs from contaminated areas into body systems through inhalation, which could easily cause common colds, flu, pneumonia, and more. Also, vaccines like flu shots should be taken annually alongside pneumococcal immunizations because they play significant roles in safeguarding against diseases that interfere with breathing processes.

Environmental Awareness

Avoidance strategy works best when dealing with pollutants allergens, and irritants. We need to be informed on how to protect ourselves against air pollution.

Respiratory Health Challenges

It is common for our respiratory health to be undermined by various infections that affect the lungs and airways. Thankfully, early identification and control of such conditions can be achieved through understanding them.

Asthma

Bronchial asthma is a persistent respiratory system ailment that is characterized by swelling of the air passages as well as their subsequent narrowing, which leads to difficulty in breathing. Some of its symptoms are shortness of breath, wheezing (a whistling sound while breathing), chest tightness, and coughing. These manifestations may be caused by triggers such as allergens, respiratory infections, exercise, cold air exposure or even emotional stress.

Management usually involves avoiding triggers, using inhaled corticosteroids to reduce inflammation and bronchodilators which relax muscles around air passage. Proper management allows individuals to live active lives without being limited by their condition.

Pneumonia

This infection occurs when there is inflammation within or both lungs, causing them to fill up with pus fluids causing coughing out of yellowish-green color phlegm, fever, chills difficulty breathing, and other signs. Several agents can cause it, including bacteria viruses, and fungi, and severity varies from mild to extreme.

Medication will be determined by the cause of pneumonia. They can include antibiotics, antiviral drugs, and fungicides. Supportive care like rest, fluid intake, and over-the-counter drugs for symptom relief, can be used as well.

Chronic Obstructive Pulmonary Disease

COPD is defined as a set of lung diseases characterized by airflow blockage and breathing disorders that include emphysema, and chronic bronchitis. Chronic cough, mucus production, shortness of breath, frequent episodes of respiratory infections, and always feeling tired. The main risk factor of COPD is smoking, but it can also result from long-term exposure to air pollutants, fumes, dust, and industrial pollution.

Thus, the management of COPD entails the amelioration of symptoms and reduction of the rate of disease progression. Bronchodilators, inhaled steroids, oxygen therapy, and pulmonary rehabilitation can be used, among others. Smoking cessation is one of the most significant interventions for preventing and treating exacerbation of COPD and enhancing the patient's quality of life.

Lung Cancer

This disease ranks among the top killers worldwide due to cancer. It comes about when abnormal cells found within the lungs grow without control, thus forming tumors which interfere with normal activities. It leads to various signs depending on where they are situated. These may include persistently coughing up blood, chest pains, shortness of breath and weight loss that cannot be explained.

When dealing with cancer, one has several options. Based on the stage and type of cancer, health professionals may recommend surgery, radiation therapy, chemotherapy, targeted treatment, or immunotherapy. Early detection through screening can enhance the chances of recovery and prolong survival rates.

We've been looking at the ways we breathe and what happens when it goes wrong. But now it's time to visit a different system altogether: the digestive system. You could think of this as the fuel tank for your body. Just as your car needs petrol, so do all the cells that make you up. We're going to find out how food gets turned into energy, which is much more exciting than it sounds!

THE DIGESTIVE SYSTEM

The digestive system. It's where every meal you've ever eaten ends up—winding its way through a fascinating network of organs and processes. Here, bites of food are transformed by our bodies into energy that keeps us going day after day.

From the moment you take your first mouthful, every organ and enzyme in this system works like a team of expert chefs to break down meals into their building blocks. It is an example of biological engineering at its best; quietly working behind the scenes so that nothing goes wasted when you eat.

Most people think digestion starts when they put something in their mouth and ends when it comes out the other end, but this tour will show you otherwise! You'll find out how taste, smell, and even seeing food can cause lots of things to happen inside you that get digestion off on the right foot. Prepare yourself for a whole new level appreciation the next time you enjoy a meal. Clinical Psychologist, Barbara Bolen, puts it best when she wrote on the topic:

> Like most things related to our bodies, we only pay attention to our digestive system when it's giving us a problem. Otherwise, we tend to overlook it and put all sorts of things into it without a second thought. Although we learn about the process of digestion in high school, most of us had other things on our minds back then. But knowing how your digestive system is supposed to work can help tremendously in terms of overall digestive health—knowledge which can help you take better care of your digestive system, more quickly identify any possible digestive problems, and help you to communicate more effectively with your healthcare provider (Bolen, 2015, para. 1)

This clearly means there's no time to waste! Let's get right to it.

Digestive Tract Anatomy

The digestive system, otherwise called the gastrointestinal (GI) tract, is an intricate and well-organized system that processes food, absorbs nutrients and eliminates waste—a complete job from start to finish. This extraordinary expedition officially starts in the mouth and proceeds through specialized organs with each one of them performing a crucial function in digestion.

Mouth

The first segment of the digestive system is commonly known as the mouth. The mouth carries out both mechanical and chemical digestion. Food that comes into the buccal cavity gets broken down into small pieces through chewing by teeth which are aided by the jaw. This process is called mastication. Have you ever thought about saliva, where it comes from and why it just keeps on coming whenever you need it? Well, take this in. Saliva is produced by salivary glands, and it moistens the food we eat (especially if its dry an needs of moisture), making it easy to swallow. Also, in saliva there is an enzyme called amylase which initiates the chemical breakdown of starches. The tongue mixes the food with this saliva, forming a round mass known as bolus that is ready for swallowing.

Esophagus

The esophagus is a muscular pipe-like structure connecting the pharynx (throat) to the stomach. It leads food from the throat to stomach where it can be digested. Peristalsis involves wave-like contractions and relaxation of muscles that push food along the esophagus towards stomach. Normally rhythmical contractions force these contents downwards; hence peristalsis acts like conveyor belt propelling them down into our bellies. The lower esophageal sphincter (LES), found at lower end of esophagus, opens up, allowing the balus entry into the stomach, but then shuts so as to prevent acid reflux or heartburn, when gastric juices flow back up toward the esophageal lining.

Stomach

The stomach is an important part of the digestive system situated on the left side below the diaphragm, between the liver and spleen. Gastric juices combine with food in this organ, resulting in the production of semi-liquid matter called chyme or pulp through a mixing action caused by muscular walls' contraction and relaxation. Digestive enzymes such as pepsin hydrochloric acid components are secreted here, too, from certain cells in the stomach lining to aid with protein digestion. Pepsin creates an acidic environment that helps break down food and kill harmful bacteria. It takes charge of the digestion of proteins into smaller peptides.

There are three regions namely: the upper part (fundus), middle portion (body) and lower segment (antrum or pyloric part), which opens into the small intestine. The opening of chyme from stomach into duodenum is controlled by a valve known as pyloric sphincter located at the junction between these two parts. Additionally, the stomach has also got another function where it contracts rhythmically, thus further mixing contents with gastric juices. This process helps in breaking down food particles, making their surface area larger for easier absorption of nutrients into the bloodstream.

Small Intestine

You might have thought this was the role of the stomach—an imagined internal pit that food and water fall into—but the small intestine is a long, coiled tube where most of the digestion and absorption of food take place. It has three divisions that we'll get into shortly: the duodenum, jejunum, and ileum.

Duodenum

Being the first part of the small intestine, it receives chyme from the stomach together with bile, which comes from the liver or gallbladder. Pancreatic juices come from the pancreas. Bile helps in emulsification of fats, making them smaller for easy digestion, while carbohydrates, proteins, and fats are further broken down by pancreatic enzymes.

Jejunum

At the center of the small intestines, this is where majority nutrient absorption takes place. It has villi and microvilli on its walls which increase its surface area for absorption. Nutrients are absorbed into the bloodstream through intestinal walls, then transported to various parts of body through blood vessels.

Ileum

This is the last, but by no means least, section of the small intestine. It is like the clean up and recycling crew, responsible for absorbing any left-over nutrients and bile acids, which are then returned back to liver so that they can be used again. Peyer's patches found here also function as clusters of lymphatic tissue meant to guard against disease-causing organisms.

Large Intestines

The large intestines, also known as the colon, absorb water and electrolytes from undigested food substances, forming solid waste (stool). Additionally, it harbors numerous friendly bacteria that help breakdown specific compounds, along with making vitamins such as vitamin K among others and safeguarding against harmful pathogens. It is comprised of:

Cecum

As soon as chyme leaves the ileum, it gets into the cecum, which happens to be the first part of the large intestine. Attached to the cecum is the appendix–this is a little finger-like projection important in immunity.

Colon

The colon is divided into four segments: ascending, transverse, descending, and sigmoid parts. While passing through these sections, chyme loses water and electrolytes, hence compacting the rest of materials into feces.

Rectum and Anus

The rectum serves as the final part of the large intestine where feces remain until they are pushed out via the anus during defecation. The anus has two sphincters–internal and external-which perform the role of regulating stool release.

Digestive Process

It all begins with eating. The moment you take a bite of your favorite meal is when the process commences. Your teeth serve to break down what you have ingested into smaller pieces, and, at the same time, your saliva begins its work of chemical digestion, thereby making it soft enough for you to swallow as it now becomes a bolus.

Once swallowed, this motionless mass travels down through your food pipe (esophagus) until it reaches the stomach where most digestion occurs. In there, powerful acids mixed with enzymes break down proteins more effectively than any other part of our system could do them justice, turning everything into chyme—a semi-liquid substance. The walls continuously churn this mixture around in order to ensure thoroughness before moving on to the next stage.

The next destination that chyme finds itself in happens to be the small intestine, which serves as the absorption champion among all the other players involved so far. It is here where pancreatic digestive juices together with bile from the liver get mixed up with what was once your lunch or dinner, breaking them down further still into fats, proteins, and carbohydrates. Their basic building blocks are then absorbed into the bloodstream through millions upon millions of finger-like projections called villi that line its inner surface. This is how the body gets minerals, vitamins, and the energy necessary for proper functioning.

After maximum uptake has taken place by various nutrients, leaving waste products behind, these undigested parts move on into the large intestine or the colon, which mainly deals with the re-absorption of water electrolytes needed elsewhere within us.

Accessory Organs

Although food does not pass through them directly, accessory organs are important in the digestive system. These are the liver, which manufactures bile; the gallbladder, which stores this bile and later secrets it into the small intestine where it emulsifies fats; and the pancreas, which produces digestive enzymes and bicarbonate that neutralizes stomach acid and breaks down carbohydrates, proteins, and fats. These organs work invisibly to aid digestion so that nutrients can be effectively broken down and absorbed. They support other digestive organs so as to keep our bodies healthy and running well.

Common Digestive Disorders

Digestive diseases and disorders are among the numerous ways we can be hindered in executing our daily activities due to the discomfort they bring or the adverse health consequences they may cause. Identifying the common ailments is important in order to administer suitable solutions.

Irritable Bowel Syndrome (IBS)

It is common for a condition called IBS to affect the colon. This can lead to symptoms including cramping, abdominal pain, bloating, gas, diarrhea, and constipation. What causes this condition remains unclear, but it can be controlled through dietary changes, stress reduction techniques, and medications. Additionally, eating foods with high fiber content, taking in enough fluids, and doing regular exercise may relieve some of its symptoms.

Gastroesophageal Reflux Disease (GERD)

When stomach acid flows back into the esophagus repeatedly, it irritates the lining. This can cause heartburn, regurgitation, and discomfort. To manage GERD, spicy foods should be avoided, and smaller meals consumed more frequently. You should also practice not lying down immediately after eating. Medication or surgery may sometimes be required to relieve symptoms and prevent further complications.

Gallstones

Sometimes referred to as biliary calculi stones, these are usually made up mainly of cholesterol or bilirubin which form in the gall-bladder and can obstruct bile ducts, leading to pain, nausea, vomiting, dyspepsia, and more. Treatment options include medications for dissolving them, surgical removal (cholecystectomy) may also be performed where necessary, or eating a low fat balanced diet so as not to expose oneself to risk getting new ones again in the future.

Constipation

This is characterized by infrequent difficult bowel movements characterized by hard dry stool often due to low fiber diet, lack of physical activity, dehydration, and certain medications. A person can gain much-needed relief by increasing their intake of nature's laxatives, like certain fruits, vegetables, whole grains, and legumes, drinking enough fluids, exercising at least three times weekly, and using over-the-counter drugs specifically manufactured for this purpose that are both safe and effective when applied correctly.

Crohn's Disease

Crohn's disease is an incurable chronic IBD that can involve any part of the gastrointestinal tract, causing intense inflammation as well as soreness accompanied with diarrhea, loss of weight, and malnutrition. Although it cannot be cured permanently, anti-inflammatory drugs such as immunosuppressants or sometimes surgery may be used to alleviate symptoms and increase quality of life for patients. It is also important that people eat balanced diets designed specifically for them.

As we wrap up here at the digestive system, it's undeniable that our bodies are equipped with an incredible and complex network of skilled professionals that transform the simple act of eating into life-sustaining energy and nutrients. Up next is the urinary system.

THE URINARY SYSTEM

Our tour is moving along smoothly, and it's now time to meet the body's sanitation staff: the urinary system. Just think about a team of really good janitors who never stop cleaning up after themselves. The best of the best. This system cleans out all the impurities from your body and maintains your health. From the adjoined twin master chemists, the kidneys, to the trusty storage tank, the bladder, it's time to learn what makes your body flush and freshen up. It may not be glamorous or even seem very important, but it sure is necessary. Here's how Byram's Healthcare explains it with a little tidbit at the end:

> The urinary system allows your body to successfully filter out your blood, creates urine as a waste product, then stores and excretes it. But that's not all it does. The urinary tract system is an integral part of your body's overall maintenance as it works to maintain homeostasis and produce necessary hormones (*Byram Healthcare*, 2019, para. 11)

Hop on, and let's get to exploring!

Kidney Function and Structure

The kidneys are important in the urinary system. The filtering of blood and elimination of waste is made possible by these bean-shaped body parts. They are located on each side of the spine beneath the ribcage. Every kidney consists of numerous small units called nephrons which aid in purifying the blood. Later, this filtered waste is converted into urine and transported to the bladder where it is stored until urination takes place. Such a necessary operation guarantees our bodies' equilibrium remains intact by keeping away poisonous materials from it. Let's now get into a more detailed overview of what our kidneys are usually up to.

Filtration and Urine Production

The kidneys' job of filtration, reabsorption, secretion, and excretion, when done well, makes certain that our body stays in prime shape. If this organ does not function optimally, this may be a disaster to the entire system. Here's what the mechanisms of filtration and urine production look like:

Filtration

The functional units of the kidney are the nephrons, wherein filtration takes place. Each kidney has massive capacity and holds around one million nephrons. These have the ability to filter blood and create urine. Filtration commences in a small network of capillaries called the glomerulus, enclosed in a cup-like structure known as Bowman's capsule.

While passing through the glomerulus, blood is subjected to high pressure, forcing water, ions, glucose, amino acids, and waste products out of it into the Bowman's capsule. This filtered fluid is known as glomerular filtrate. These smaller molecules pass through the glomerular membrane while larger molecules like proteins and blood cells remain in the blood stream. It is this selective filtration that helps maintain proper balance of substances in the body.

Reabsorption

When glomerular filtrate enters the renal tubule, reabsorption begins. Several segments make up the renal tubule: the proximal convoluted tubule, loop of Henle, distal convoluted tubule, and collecting duct. Every one of these segments has a special function of carrying substances back into the blood.

- Proximal Convoluted Tubule

Here, 99% of water, glucose, amino-acids, and associated ions—like sodium and potassium—are reabsorbed from the filtrate. This reabsorption is aided by the process of passive diffusion as well as by active transport.

- Loop of Henle

The loop of Henle is divided into a descending limb and ascending limb. Since the medulla (the inner part of the organ) has high osmolarity (concentration of solute particles), more water diffuses from its lumen to surrounding capillaries. The ascending limb, on the other hand, does not allow water movement but transports sodium and chlorine ions out of the filtrate, further concentrating the urine.

- Distal Convoluted Tubule

This segment fine-tunes reabsorption of sodium, potassium, and calcium, which are regulated by aldosterone and parathyroid hormones, for instance. Here also water is reabsorbed depending on the presence or absence of antidiuretic hormone (ADH).

- Collecting Duct

Final adjustment of urine concentration occurs in the collecting duct. Water can be absorbed more under the influence of ADH, resulting to concentrated urine. If ADH levels fall, then less water is reabsorbed leading to dilute urine.

Secretion

On one hand, while reabsorption gets back essential substances, secretion transports additional waste products, toxins, and excess ions from the blood into the renal tubule. This takes place mainly in distal convoluted tubule and collecting ducts. Purification of the blood as well as maintenance of an acid-base balance is facilitated through secretion.

Urine Formation

By the time filtrate reaches the end of the collecting duct, it will have become urine. The final urinary composition consists mostly of urea, creatinine, and uric acid, along with waste products, such as extra ions and water, substances that are not needed by the body.

Thereafter, this urine flows into the renal pelvis that channels it to the ureter.

Storage and Excretion

The ureters in the kidney connect to the bladder where urine is stored until excretion. Having a storage capacity of about 400-600 millimeters of urine, when the bladder fills, one feels the need to urinate because there are stretch receptors that are located on the walls of this organ. Urination finally takes place only in a state of relaxation, when both internal and external urethral sphincters relax, and only the bladder contracts, forcing urine out via urethra.

Urinary Tract Anatomy

This intricate network includes four major parts: kidneys, ureters (tubes connecting kidneys with bladder), the bladder itself (which acts as a reservoir for large volumes of fluids), and the urethra, where urine exits during urination process.

Ureters

Thin, muscular tubes known as ureters whisk away urine from the renal pelvis right over to the bladder. They are around 10-12 inches long. Kidneys use rhythmic contractions referred to as peristalsis to help push urine down through narrow the passageways of these two ducts, leading into the bladder until release.

Bladder

There is a bladder in the pelvis. It is a hollow, muscular sac that stores urine temporarily. Its walls are made of detrusor muscle, which allows for expansion and contraction. When it is empty, it looks like a deflated balloon, but it can hold up to 400-600 milliliters comfortably.

As the bladder fills with liquid waste products from our body called urine, stretch receptors on its wall send messages to our brain so we feel the urge to go "pee". The internal urethral sphincter keeps closed off, preventing an opening into the external world until we decide when and where this should happen. We can do this voluntarily by using external control of muscles around the opening of the tube leading outside called the urethra.

Urethra

This is the passage for urine where it leaves body, called the urethra. Males and females have different lengths and functions of this tube-like structure. In females, it measures approximately 1.5 to 2 inches long, opening just above vaginal entrance. The male's extends about 8 inches, passing through the prostate gland and penis, serving also as the conduit for semen during ejaculation.

Urination, known as micturition, commences by the contraction of muscles in the bladder and the opening of the internal urethral sphincter in response to brain signals. Simultaneously with this action, we deliberately release tension in our exterior urethral sphincter, thus enabling urine to pass through the urethra. It is this harmony that guarantees speedy removal of waste products from our bodies.

Urinary Health and Disorders

When the urinary system fails, it causes a variety of issues that reduce the quality of life we experience. The urinary system can be affected by many disorders that may present themselves through slight discomfort or severe pain and other health problems. Here are a few common disorders associated with the urinary system:

Urinary Tract Infections (UTIs)

Bacteria may infect any part of the kidneys, but usually it is the bladder or urethra. This condition is identified in a person who has a strong desire for urination, an intense burning feeling when passing urine, cloudy and bad-smelling urine, as well as pain in their lower abdomen. Urinary tract infections arise when bacteria like escherichia coli pass through the urethra into the kidneys. Women are more susceptible because they have shorter urethras than men, making these parts vulnerable to germs. Once diagnosed, doctors advise that antibiotics be taken to prevent further spread up towards to the kidneys, which would result in serious illness.

Kidney Stones

Solid mineral salts termed "stones" sometimes form within the kidneys, blocking the ureters and causing severe agony, especially while passing them out. Symptoms comprise sharp back/side aches, painful urination, pinkish-brownish urine, and nauseous feelings. Various factors raise the chance of developing kidney stones: dehydration, certain diets, obesity, or it can simply be heredity. As such, treatment may involve managing the sufferer's pain level through drugs and increasing fluid intake either naturally or by surgeries designed to break the stones apart, removing those fragments completely from the body.

Chronic Renal Disease (CKD)

CKD is a state where the kidneys lose function slowly over time. It may be caused by diabetes, hypertension, or glomerulonephritis, or other reasons. Symptoms will not show until later stages, and they include tiredness, swollen legs or ankles, frequent urination at night, and high blood pressure. Management involves treating underlying conditions with medications and, when necessary, dialysis or kidney transplant.

Bladder Disorders

Interstitial cystitis as well as bladder cancer are bladder problems. They can lead to chronic pain, frequent urination, and blood in urine. With no known cause, interstitial cystitis is a continuous condition that causes pressure or pain in the bladder. Another disorder is bladder cancer, which refers to malignant cells growing within the lining of the bladder wall. For both, early detection coupled with proper treatment goes a long way in helping manage these conditions effectively.

Though it might not seem like it at first because they deal with the dirty work, it's clear that the urinary system is one of the body's unsung heroes that works tirelessly to keep our bodies functioning smoothly. We should do our best to keep it running as smoothly as possible. Next, we'll explore another fascinating aspect of our anatomy—the endocrine system—revealing more about all that goes on back stage to keep us alive.

THE ENDOCRINE SYSTEM

While the endocrine system may not boast the fame of the digestive or respiratory systems, pay this no mind. This "bad boy" serves as a crucial means of overall well-being. It does so by working in incognito mode to ensure all growth processes are well taken care of. The glands of the endocrine system—pituitary, thyroid, adrenal glands, and some others—release hormones directly into the bloodstream. These chemicals travel around delivering instructions on how things should be done; they help control things such as growth or even mood while at it. Every gland has its own duties and specific types of hormones it produces, but together these make up part and parcel of this system, forming one whole cohesive unit responsible for keeping the internal environment in check.

Let's uncover the secrets of this behind-the-scenes system and how it keeps our bodies going like clockwork.

Major Endocrine Glands

Endocrine system is made up of important glands, each with its unique tasks and hormones. These work together to keep different body functions under control so that everything moves as it should. Let's take a closer look at these major endocrine parts and what they do.

Pituitary Glands

Gaining its nickname from its small size and location at the base of the brain, the pituitary gland is commonly known as the "master gland." Despite its diminutive stature, it produces numerous hormones that regulate various bodily functions.

Comprising two main parts—namely, anterior and posterior portions—this gland secretes growth hormones responsible for promoting cell production: the adrenocorticotropic hormone stimulates cortisol secretion by adrenal glands, along with the thyroid-stimulating hormone that is essential in inducing thyroid hormonal activity, and more. Meanwhile, the posterior part secretes hypothalamus-produced antidiuretic hormones, which help maintain water balance in our bodies. It also secretes oxytocin—crucial during childbirth and lactation—storing them within its confines until required by surrounding tissues or organs.

Thyroid Gland

You'll find a butterfly-shaped thyroid gland under the Adam's Apple in the neck. This gland makes hormones that control how fast our body works, our energy levels, and how we grow. The hormones responsible for this are released by the thyroid and kind of sound like dinosaurs: triiodothyronine and thyroxine. These hormones affect how we burn calories, which in turn impacts every cell, tissue, and organ in our body. Additionally, calcitonin—another hormone generated from this gland—helps regulate blood calcium levels by preventing its discharge from bones.

Parathyroid Glands

On the back of the thyroid gland, sit four little parathyroid glands. They are behind each side of your thyroid gland and help to keep calcium levels balanced in our body. They increase blood calcium levels by releasing calcium from bone stimulating osteoclast activity, enhancing intestinal calcium absorption and decreasing calcium excretion in the urine.

Adrenal Glands

On top of each kidney are the triangular-shaped adrenal glands. These glands produce many hormones that help in responding to stress, metabolism control, immune function, and other processes. Corticosteroids (including cortisol) that can control metabolism and responses to stress are produced by the cortex, the outer part of adrenal gland. Aldosterone is another important hormone released, which controls sodium-potassium levels, therefore affecting the regulation of blood pressure. The inner part, known as the medulla, produces catecholamines like adrenaline (epinephrine) and noradrenaline (norepinephrine). These prepare body for a "fight or flight" situation when there is stress.

Pancreas

Have you heard of the pancreas before? You probably have. It's nestled behind the stomach, and it serves both endocrine and exocrine functions. It plays an important role in regulating blood sugar levels and more. By diffusing glucose into cells, it supports energy production.

Gonads

The primary reproductive glands consist of the testes found in males and ovaries found in females. They are both called gonads. These are involved in the reproduction process, though not essential for survival. Ovaries are positioned within the pelvic cavity in women and produce estrogen and progesterone that regulate menstrual cycle. These hormones also regulate the reproductive system's development and other sexual characteristics like breast growth. Males, on the other hand, have their testes situated outside their abdomen within the scrotum. There they generate the testosterone responsible for sperm production, muscle mass accumulation, increased bone density, and secondary sexual traits such as beard and voice changes.

Pineal Gland

There is a small pinecone-shaped organ known as the pineal gland deep inside our head that releases melatonin, enabling us to sleep well at night. This hormone acts on our circadian rhythms by causing alertness during daytime hours while promoting sleep at night time, thereby serving as a natural synchronizer of our sleep/wake cycles.

Thymus

The thymus is situated just behind the sternum in the upper chest. It is most active during childhood and adolescence when it makes significant contributions to immune functions. These hormones include thymosins thatpromote T cell maturation and differentiation, which are vital for adaptive immunity.

Hormones and Their Functions

Our health relies on hormones. They act as internal regulators of the body by ensuring various systems work together. Endocrine glands release chemical messengers that coordinate growth, metabolism, reproduction, and stress response among many other things. For example, the hormone responsible for growth also repairs tissues, while our energy levels and metabolism are controlled by thyroid hormones. Insulin prevents diabetes mellitus through its regulation of blood sugar levels, and cortisol aids in managing stress. Sexual development and fertility are brought about by estrogens, progesterone, and testosterone, which also regulate sleep through melatonin for a well-balanced sleep/wake cycle.

Our systems would be in chaos without these hormones. Growth might not occur, or it could be stunted completely; energy levels may become too low one moment then too high the next; blood sugar might rise to dangerous levels at times. Added to this, we may not only fail to react appropriately towards stressful situations but also our reproductive functions could shut down; sleeping patterns could become irregular, and bones could weaken due to disturbed calcium homeostasis. Each hormone is uniquely essential in maintaining internal stability while enhancing overall healthiness. Together, they all work together toward this end. They allow us to adjust accordingly to changes in the environment with the ability to heal injuries. The absence of any one hormone disrupts this delicate balance, thereby emphasizing their important function in our daily life.

Endocrine Disorders

Health issues may be caused by the glands generating too many or too few hormones, these are called endocrine disorders. Diabetes is among the common problems, whereby insulin is not produced in enough amount by the pancreas, or it fails to work properly within the body, leading to high levels of sugar in blood. There is also hypothyroidism that refers to an abnormality of low activity exhibited when little thyroxine (T4) and triiodothyronine (T3) hormones are secreted from thyroid glands. It results in fatigue, depression, weight gain, and other conditions, while hyperthyroidism is excessive production of these two types of hormones, causing rapid heartbeats coupled with weight loss and anxiety.

Addison's disease is another adrenal disorder that results from insufficient cortisol production, resulting in fatigue, muscle weakness, and low blood pressure. Whereas Cushing's syndrome, caused by excess cortisol, leads to weight gain, high blood pressure, and osteoporosis. Polycystic ovarian syndrome (PCOS) is another disorder that causes hormonal imbalances, affecting menstrual periods and fertility. Disorders related to the pituitary gland can be associated with growth hormone deficit, causing growth abnormalities in children or acromegaly, characterized by the abnormal growth of hands and feet among adults.

These disorders show that hormonal equilibrium is important as well as taking good care of the endocrine system. Treatment usually encompasses hormone replacement therapy, drugs commonly used for rehabilitation purposes, lifestyle changes, and consistent monitoring towards regaining optimal health.

We're almost at the end of the body's tour. Up next are the lymphatic and immune systems. I can't wait to learn the exciting nuggets awaiting us at this stop.

THE LYMPHATIC AND IMMUNE SYSTEMS

Imagine that while gardening you get a slight cut on your hand. It may appear minor at first sight, but it is actually a small breach in your skin for bacteria and other pathogens to enter the body. This is where the lymphatic and immune systems come in.

Upon entering the wound, bacteria start to multiply. Almost immediately there are neutrophils, which are referred to as immune system's first responders. These white blood cells are part of the innate immunity that provides rapid response though not specific to invaders. They engage bacteria in order to limit infection.

At the same time, the lymphatic system starts functioning. Lymphatic vessels surrounding a wound absorb extra fluid, germs, and dead cells, then escort them into nearby lymph nodes. These act like sieves catching injurious particles and offer an area for immune cells to interact with pathogens.

Within these nodes of lymphocytes, defense functions such as B-cells take over and produce antibodies, which are a type of protein that identifies and neutralizes bacteria. Meanwhile, T-cells can either kill infected cells or facilitate this for other cells through immune response coordination.

This is the way our lymphatic and immune system work. They work together to limit or neutralize harmful invaders in the body.

Lymphatic System Anatomy

To maintain the fluid balance of our bodies, fight infections, and help us digest fats, we have an elaborate lymphatic system. Sometimes, this system is not given enough credit for its importance, but we'll give you a closer look at what it does to begin changing the tide.

Lymph and Lymph Vessels

The lymphatic system is an intricate web that carries a transparent liquid called lymph. It is derived from the interstitial fluid found in body tissues and cells. Nutrients, oxygen, and waste products are carried by it. When blood passes through capillaries, some of its plasma seeps into the tissue, forming what we call as the interstitial fluid. Mostly, this gets reabsorbed by capillaries, but those that don't enter the lymphatic vessels as lymph.

These lymphatic capillaries are like blood vessels, but they belong to a different kind of circulatory system where everything flows in one direction toward our hearts instead. These start off as tiny dead-end capillaries throughout the body, especially in tissue near skin and mucous membranes. Lymphatic capillaries join up to form bigger lymphatics, which have valves to prevent lymph back flow. Gradually, these vessels converge until two major ducts form: the right lymphatic duct and thoracic duct. The first drains from the right arm, right head side and right chest, emptying into subclavian vein on the right while the thoracic duct empties into the left subclavian vein after draining from all other parts of the body.

Lymph Nodes

Now, on to lymph nodes. These are distributed throughout the lymphatic vessels, and they appear as bean-shaped structures. They act as strainers that hold impurities such as bacteria, viruses, and cancer cells. The immune system's major players can be found in each lymph node, including T cells, B cells (these are types of lymphocytes), and macrophages that rid the body of these invaders.

The afferent lymphatic vessels (tubes that carry lymph fluid into lymph nodes) drain into the node, forcing the lymph through its sinuses. The immune cells within the node scrutinize this fluid for any indications of pathogens. In case there are identified pathogens, an immune response is triggered. If an infection by pathogens is detected, the resulting immunity leads to multiplication and activation of T and B-lymphocytes. Then efferent lymphatic vessels drain filtered lymph from the node directing it towards heart.

Primary Lymphatic Organs

The lymphatic system is made up of the primary lymphatic organs where the T and B cells are formed and mature. These are the bone marrow and thymus.

Bone Marrow

The bone marrow can be found in the cavities of our bones. It is actually where all blood-cell elements, including lymphocytes (B-cells), develop. It is in the bone marrow that immature T cells migrate from to secondary lymphoid organs.

Thymus

Just as we learned that the thymus has endocrine function, it also has lymphatic function. We've established that it is a butterfly-shaped gland that lies behind the sternum, at the level above the heart. It is here that T cells develop into their final form. It plays a big role developing a functional and self-tolerant T-cell repertoire.

Secondary Lymphatic Organs

These are sites where mature lymphocytes become activated and mount an immune response called secondary lymphoid organs. They include lymph nodes, spleen, tonsils, and mucosal-associated lymphoid tissue (MALT).

Spleen

Located in the upper left abdomen, it filters out old or damaged red blood cells as well as pathogens from the blood. It also helps store blood, many macrophages, and a large numbers of white blood cells.

Tonsils

Located at back of throat, they are collection points for several clusters of lymphatic nodules which prevent or protect our body against pathogenic agents that we inhale or swallow. For instance, when one gets sick with colds or flu, these parts get inflamed, making them sore.

Mucosa-Associated Lymphoid Tissue (MALT)

MALT includes aggregate follicles in regions such as the stomach wall lining and bronchial walls, while others occur in regions like the appendixes or Peyer's patches along the small intestine. These tissues are a primary line of defense against mucosal pathogens that gain access into the body.

Lymph Circulation

Finally, there are several mechanisms that keep the flow of lymph through the lymphatic system. Skeletal muscles during movement help in moving lymph through the vessels. Furthermore, the smooth muscles present in the walls of lymphatic vessels contract rhythmically, while breathing causes a change in pressure within the thoracic cavity, a factor that also facilitates lymph flow.

Immune Response Mechanisms

Our immune system is a surveillance network on constant lookout for foreign pathogens like bacteria, viruses, and other invaders that it protects us from. This is achieved through the two primary mechanisms called innate immunity and adaptive immunity. Both play distinct but complementary roles in maintaining good health. So, let's get into the captivating workings behind these immune responses.

Innate Immunity

Innate immunity—like a frontline soldier in an uncertain war—serves as the first line of defense for the body against pathogens. It is indiscriminate, meaning it does not target or prioritize specific invaders, but reacts in a general way, impartially, across a wide range of threats. This system responds upon completion of detection, instantly, since it is always active.

The first parts of innate immunity include physical and chemical barriers that prevent entry of pathogens into the body. The largest organ that we have, the skin, acts as a physical barrier, while the respiratory, digestive, and genitourinary tracts contain mucus membranes which trap pathogenic microorganisms before they can cause damage. Chemical barriers include stomach acid, which kills any pathogens taken in. Saliva and tears possess enzymes that break down bacterial cell walls.

When pathogens manage to bypass these barriers, cellular defenses come into play. Key players in this response include phagocytes (such as macrophages and neutrophils) and natural killer (NK) cells.

If pathogens make it past these sieves, they face cellular defenses. The main players in this response are phagocytes (macrophages and available neutrophils) as well as certain subpopulations of cells like NK Cells.

Phagocytosis

White blood cells known as macrophages and neutrophil cells engulf pathogens by digesting them. Macrophages also release vesicles filled with cytokines, which are signaling molecules for other immune cells to come at infection site leading to inflammation.

Natural Killer Cells

NK cells have a unique ability of identifying infected target host cells as well as malignant tumor targets because they release perforin molecules, which trigger apoptosis (the process of programmed cell death, allowing the body to remove unwanted or damaged cells).

Role of White Blood Cells (WBC)

In the immune system, WBCs, otherwise called leukocytes, are very important to combat infections as well as other foreign bodies. We've touched on some of their roles earlier on, like macrophages and neutrophils, which surround pathogens, and we've established that adaptive immunity revolves around B-cells and T-cells.

Immune System Disorders

The immune system is the body's defense line against diseases and infections. Even so, it sometimes malfunctions, giving rise to disorders of the immune system. These disorders can come from hyperactive immune responses, anemia immune response, or autoreactive anemia, where a person's own tissues are attacked by the body itself. There are several major types of immune system disorders.

Psoriasis

Psoriasis is an autoimmune condition that is long-term and affects the skin primarily. The disease makes cells on the top layer of the skin multiply faster than normal—up to 10 times faster—and leads to red patches covered with scales, which may be dry and itchy. Over-active inflammation and rapid production of skin cells provoke this immunological reaction leading to patches on certain parts like knees, elbows, scalp, and lower back. Topical treatments are available along with phototherapy or systemic medications which suppress immunity.

Graves' Disease

Graves' disease is an autoimmune disorder characterized by overproduction of thyroid hormones (hyperthyroidism) from the thyroid gland. Symptoms include weight loss, increased heart rate, nervousness, tremors, and bulging eyes (exophthalmos). Our immune systems will mistakenly attack this gland making it become over active. Antithyroid drugs might be used while for others radioactive iodine therapy or surgery might be done in part or all of our thyroid glands.

Alopecia Areata

Round patches of hair loss on the scalp, face, or other areas of the body are a symptom of alopecia areata, which is an autoimmune condition. The immune system turns against the follicles, resulting in hair shedding. Though not known for sure, it is believed that genetic factors and environmental conditions may be the cause. This hair fall can happen suddenly and without warning, but it is not life threatening. Treatment options include corticosteroids, topical immunotherapy, and minoxidil, although re-growth varies.

Vitiligo

Vitiligo is an autoimmune disease that causes depigmentation or permanent loss of skin coloration from certain areas of the body. Melanocytes, which produce melanin, the pigment responsible for skin coloration, are attacked by immune cells. This gives rise to white spots on different parts of the body surface. Vitiligo might not harm a person's health or spread to others; however, it can affect one's physical look and self-esteem negatively. Treatments involve using corticosteroid creams applied topically, light therapy such as UVB excimer laser treatment, and skin grafting depending on individual cases.

Hashimoto's Thyroiditis

When the immune system destroys the thyroid gland, this disorder is called Hashimoto's thyroiditis. It causes an underactive thyroid or hypothyroidism. Inadequate production of hormones is characteristic of this disorder, and it results in fatigue, increase in weight, cold intolerance, depression, and dry skin. Hormone replacement therapy is usually administered during treatment to correct the levels of normal thyroid hormone.

We're now in a better position to appreciate how tough our bodies are as well as how intricate they can be.

Now, we head on to our last stop where we will look at another integral system that affects our overall health and, amazingly, the continuance of the human race. Let's keep going. The incredible world of the reproductive systems awaits!

The Reproductive System

The reproductive system is often a subject of curiosity, fascination, and sometimes embarrassment. It's surrounded by many myths and misconceptions, but it plays an irreplaceable role in keeping life going forward. There are common views about the reproductive system, on topics including the miracle of creating new life, puberty changes, and the challenges and adversities associated with life thereafter.

One popular myth is that the reproductive system only becomes active at certain stages of life such as puberty or when one is pregnant. However, the truth is, that it is always working, controlling hormones, maintaining reproductive health, and preparing for the possibility of new life. Another prominent myth on this issue concerns conception, and that fertility alone constitutes reproductive health. The fact is, that reproductive health includes more than fertility. That aspect needs to be addressed along with menstrual health, sexual health, and prevention and treatment of health challenges impacting women.

This final stop on our tour of the human body will demystify reproduction while highlighting its essential functions and significance. The male and female reproductive systems are marvels of biology designed for both creation as well as general well-being. From the ovaries and testes producing vital hormones to ovulation and spermatogenesis, each component of this complex system has a critical role.

We will explore the anatomy and physiology of reproduction organs, learning how they relate to each other functionally. We'll also look at some common conditions that can affect reproductive health, drawing attention to the importance of regular medical check-ups and a healthy lifestyle. By the time we're through at this stop, you will have comprehensively understood reproduction, appreciating its intricacy and recognizing its indispensable contributions towards human life.

Male Reproductive Anatomy

The male reproductive system is a network of organs and structures with coordinated activities to form, store, and transfer sperm;

produce hormones, and conduct other functions necessary for male reproductive health. To understand the importance of this system in reproduction and in overall health, one needs to know more about its structure.

Testes

The testes are sac-like organs hanging from the pubic region and the main reproductive organs in males. They are also called testicles. They are oval shaped and located in the scrotum, a pouch outside the stomach. This positioning is crucial because it enables them to be cooler and this helps in the production of healthy sperms.

Each testis consists of lobules, which contain seminiferous tubules where sperm production takes place, a process known as spermatogenesis. These tubules are lined with germ cells that produce sperm after undergoing division and maturation. Hormonal regulation of this process occurs through the follicle-stimulating hormone (FSH), testosterone, produced by Leydig cells located between seminiferous tubules.

Epididymis

After being formed inside seminiferous tubules, sperms move into the epididymis. This can be described as a long, coiled tube that sits on top of each testis. Sperms are stored here, maturing before they can fertilize an egg. They gain the ability to move independently during their stay here. This takes about two to four weeks for complete development. The epididymis is also involved in the process of reabsorption of excess water and the process of sperm concentration.

Vas Deferens

Ductus deferens, or vas deferens, is a muscular tube which collects developed sperm from the epididymis and takes them to ejaculatory ducts in preparation for ejaculation. During ejaculation, the smooth muscle walls of the vas deference contract, projecting sperm forward. It also serves as a place where sperm are stored up until they are ejaculated.

Seminal Vesicles

Seminal vesicles are two accessory glands lying at the back of the urinary bladder and above the prostate gland. They contribute most of the seminal fluid that make up not less than 60-70% of total fluid found in semen. The fluid contains fructose as a source of energy for sperm and other substances which boosts their motility and sustainability.

Prostate Gland

The prostate is an organ that is about the size of a walnut located below the bladder and in front of the rectum. This organ surrounds the urethra, the tube through which urine and semen are discharged outwards from the body. The prostate gland generates about 20-30% of semen's total volume in the form of milky fluid containing enzymes, prostate specific antigen (PSA), and other nourishing agents for sperm protection purposes. At ejaculation, muscles around the prostate contract, expelling its fluid into the urethra where it mingles with sperm and seminal fluids.

Bulbourethral Glands

The two Cowper's glands, which are also referred to as bulbourethral glands, are situated below the prostate gland and located one on either side of urethra. These organs secrete a watery, lubricating fluid that is discharged before ejaculation. It helps in the movement of sperm through the urethra and eliminates any acidic remains of urine, thereby providing a favorable environment for the survival of sperm.

Urethra and Penis

This is like a double-sided pipe that plays a role of passing both urine and semen. During sexual intercourse, the passage through the urethra is blocked partially to prevent the passage of urine, only permitting the semen to flow. It's like having a security guard at the door that knows who should exit when. The penis contains a canal known as the urethra on the length of its shaft that is responsible for allowing urine to exit the body during urination and through which semen is released during ejaculation.

The penis consists of three main parts: the root, body (shaft), and glans (head). The body has cylindrical masses containing erectile tissue: namely, two corpus cavernosum and one corpus spongiosum. They fill with blood at arousal, making self-erection possible. In males who have not been circumcised, there is sensitive skin covering the penis tip known as the glans.

Female Reproductive Anatomy

The female reproductive system is an intricate and highly coordinated chain of structures and organs that collectively and specifically produces ova (eggs) and ensures fertilization as well as fetal development and childbirth. This system also helps in the maintenance of hormones and the female metabolic calendar, which includes menstruation.

Ovaries

Located on either side of the uterus within the pelvic cavity, ovaries are paired glandular organs that produce eggs and secrete hormones like estrogen and progesterone. They are equivalent to the testes in males. Each ovary may contain thousands of follicles that each house an immature egg cell waiting for maturation during a menstrual cycle. During this cycle, usually one follicle becomes fully developed, leading to its release. This process is called ovulation.

Fallopian Tubes

Fallopian tubes are narrow muscular tubes, also known as uterine tubes or oviducts, that extend from upper corners of the uterus toward the ovaries. The role of the fallopian tubes primarily involves transportation of eggs from the ovary to uterus where implantation can take place if fertilization occurs. Near the ends of the fallopian tubes are the fimbriae, finger-like projections that help capture released eggs, guiding them into the tubes. When sperms meet eggs within these tubes, fertilization takes place.

Uterus

The womb or uterus is an empty, muscular organ positioned in the hips, behind the bladder and ahead of the rectum. It's shaped like a pear and has three different layers: the outer layer known as the perimetrium, the middle muscular layer called myometrium, and the inner lining or endometrium. There are two main roles that this part of a female body plays, providing protection and nourishment for developing fetuses during pregnancies and aiding their expulsion childbirth.

There are basically two sections into which the uterus can be divided, namely the corpus (body) and cervix. The former is the larger upper part where fertilized eggs get implanted to develop into babies, while the latter, being the lower, narrow region opening into the vagina, acts as a passageway through which sperms enter the uterus. Menstrual blood and babies also exit from the cervix.

Endometrium

The innermost lining of the uterus, referred to as endometrium, changes cyclically in response hormonal signals throughout menstrual cycle. During the initial half of the menstrual cycle, it thickens, becoming highly rich in blood vessels so that if there is conception pregnancy can occur. If this doesn't happen, it sheds off, leading to menstrual flow.

Cervix

The cervix is located at the vagina's lowermost point. It consists mainly of dense fibrous tissues mixed with smooth muscles. Two functions of the cervix are allowing uterine mucous membrane cells to exit through the vagina during periods and permitting sperms to gain entry into the uterus when fertilization takes place. In preparation for delivery through the birth canal, the cervix dilates, meaning that it opens up while thinning (effacing) during labor contractions.

Vagina

A tube-like structure, the vagina is made up mostly of muscles running from the cervix down towards to the external genitalia. The vagina serves several purposes. These include acting as a conduit for mensuration flow, being a receptacle for the penis during sexual intercourse, and serving as the birth canal for the baby to exit the mother's womb. Mucous lining found within the walls of the vagina keeps tissues lubricated, while its pH level remains slightly acidic, helping to protect against infections.

Vulva

Collectedly known as the vulva or the external genital organs, this reproductive body part consists of different components which safe-guard other internal reproductive system parts and facilitate a sexual stimulation sensation. The following are some main features of the vulva:

- Labia Majora: These are the outer lips that surround and protect other external genitalia.
- Labia Minora: These are the inner lips enveloping the vaginal and urethral opening.
- Clitoris: This is a very sensitive, small part situated at anterior intersection of the labium minus. It has numerous nerve endings and is a key player in sexual arousal and pleasure.
- Urethral Opening: This is the external opening of the urethra. It is situated just above the vaginal aperture where urine gets expelled during urination.
- Vaginal Opening: This is the entryway into the vagina which may partially be covered by a hymen, a thin membrane present for some individuals.

Reproductive Health and Disorders

Both the male and female reproductive systems can, at times, suffer from reproductive health issues and disorders. According to research by the National Institute of Environmental Health Sciences:

> Exposure to environmental pollutants can lead to disorders that affect the function of male and female reproductive systems. These problems can occur at any stage in life and include birth defects of the reproductive system, pregnancy complications, early puberty, developmental disorders, low birth weight, preterm birth, reduced fertility, impotence, and menstrual disorders (Reproductive System Disorders, n.d.).

Let's take a look at some of the disorders that plague both male and female reproductive systems.

Male Reproductive Disorders

Erectile Dysfunction (ED)

Erectile dysfunction is the inability for males to achieve or maintain an erection that suffices for satisfactory sexual intercourse. It may be due to many different causes, including stress from personal problems, hormonal imbalance, damage of nerves because of diabetes mellitus, or alcoholism and so forth. Treatment options include lifestyle changes such as weight loss and exercise programs, medications, counseling therapies, and even surgery in extreme cases.

BPH

Benign prostatic hyperplasia refers to a noncancerous enlargement of the prostate gland. It often leads to lower urinary tract symptoms which include hesitancy when trying to urinate, weak stream, or increased urination frequency, especially at night. The choice for treatment depends on how severe these signs are, but drugs can be given initially, followed by various surgical interventions if need arises.

Prostatitis

Prostatitis is simply inflammation involving the prostate gland. It is mainly caused by bacterial infection though other factors may also contribute toward it. Common symptoms consist of pain around the pelvis area, difficulty with urination or emptying bladder completely due to obstructed flow, and painful urination. Antibiotics are usually used for treating bacterial infections or other medications to treat the uncomfortable symptoms.

Testicular Cancer

Cancer that originates within one's testicles is what is referred to as testicular cancer. It most frequently attacks younger males between fifteen years and thirty-five years old. It presents itself with certain signs like a lump found anywhere in either testicle sack accompanied with discomfort and heavy feelings in the scrotum region. Early diagnosis together with prompt intervention, such as surgery, is effective. Radiotherapy/chemotherapy can also result in favorable outcomes.

Female Reproductive Disorders

Polycystic Ovary Syndrome

Irregular menstrual cycles, excess male hormone production, and multiple cysts on the ovaries are common symptoms of PCOS. It can also cause irregular periods or none at all, acne, hirsutism (excessive hair growth), and obesity. The menstrual cycle may be regulated with lifestyle changes alone or in combination with medication and insulin resistance treatments might also be necessary.

Endometriosis

This condition involves the growth of tissue similar to the lining of the uterus, but outside of it. It often leads to pain as well as inflammation and sometimes infertility too. Symptoms may include very painful periods, chronic pelvic pain throughout each month (not only during menstruation), and pain during or after sex, which is usually deep-seated rather than superficial. Pain relief drugs such as ibuprofen can help alleviate some discomfort but hormonal therapies as well surgical procedures targeting the removal of endometrial tissues might sometimes be needed, depending upon severity level among other factors.

Uterine Fibroids

Fibroids are benign tumors that grow in or around the womb. They sometimes cause heavy periods or discomfort such as pain or pressure symptoms like frequent urination due to their size compressing nearby structures. However, they often go unnoticed without any symptoms at all depending on their location and size. The treatment approach taken with this condition will depend largely upon whether a woman desires future childbearing potential. Treatment approaches include monitoring of the condition through regular checkups and non-steroidal anti-inflammatory options. More aggressive approaches might involve myomectomy (removal fibroid) or hysterectomy (removal entire uterus).

Ovarian Cysts

Fluid-filled pouches known as cysts can develop on or inside one (or both) ovaries. These growths are usually harmless and disappear without treatment over time, but they may produce symptoms if they rupture or become twisted, thereby causing complications. Treatment depends upon factors like size/type of cyst as well as the patient's age and general health status. Options include watchful waiting (regular monitoring), medication used to suppress ovulation temporarily, or even surgical removal in some cases.

Cervical Dysplasia and Cancer

The term cervical dysplasia refers to changes in the cells on the surface of your cervix detected through a pap smear. If left untreated, this condition can progress into cervical cancer caused by human papillomavirus (HPV) infection, which is also linked with other anogenital cancers like anal malignancies among others. Preventive measures such as vaccination against various HPV types responsible for most cases worldwide along with regular screenings. Preventative measures should be taken seriously since they help to detect precancerous lesions early when they're still easily treatable.

And there it is! The last station of our incredible tour around the human body. It has been what you may call an eventful experience, wouldn't you agree? At our last stop, we looked into every captivating aspect of the reproductive system. Put it all together and we have now seen how each and every process in our body functions perfectly with the ultimate aim of maintaining our health and ensuring our survival. I am grateful for your company in this unforgettable tour. It is my hope that you leave this experience with a newly found interest and wonder for your body. Never lose your curiosity! Go forward and, in your own way, explore the world of human anatomy further!

CONCLUSION

Corporative and inquisitive body explorers! It's been an absolute pleasure exploring the wonders of the human body with you. I was so happy to show you around, and your curiosity has made it all a very unforgettable experience.

We began our tour with the skeletal system, which is the strong framework that supports and protects us. We saw how bones, joints, and cartilage all work together to keep us upright and moving so we can do things like walk, run, and sit up straight comfortably. From long leg bones to tiny finger joints, we realized just how essential this system is for overall health.

The next area we explored was the muscular system—the body part responsible for making everything move! Learning about what makes muscles function well also gave us some tips on maintaining strength throughout life.

Then came along my favorite part, the nervous system! This, we learned, is like your body's control center. We looked at different parts such as the brain, spinal cord, and peripheral nerves, which send signals from one place to another telling the nerves what they should do. It amazed me with its intricacy because every single thing we do involves it somehow.

Next up was exploring how blood flows through our body during circulation. This includes the heart, blood vessels, and blood itself. It's not as scary as it sounded after all, as blood works as a transportation network delivering oxygen and nutrients needed by cells. We also talked about maintaining a healthy heart, because it can suffer from various cardiovascular diseases.

For some fresh air, we decided to make a stop at the respiratory system. Starting off from the nose, we traveled down to the lungs where the exchange of gases occurs. We learned so much!

One of my other favorite stops was the digestive system where food goes after being eaten, because who doesn't love food? We passed through the mouth, stomach, intestines, and more, learning how all these organs break down complex molecules into simpler ones to be absorbed by cells.

After digestion was complete, we definitely had to go! We moved to the urinary system, which is tasked with removing waste products from our bodies. Understanding this system has enabled us to know how to prevent common problems like UTIs or kidney stones.

Next up was the endocrine system, the body's chemical communication network! We learned about hormones produced by glands and their role in growth, metabolism, and mood regulation. Imbalances may have various effects on health, so, it's a good idea to ensure this system is working properly at all times.

With a stop to the lymphatic and immune systems, we were able to appreciate how our bodies defend themselves against infections. We also saw what happens when these defenses fail leading to diseases such as cancer or AIDS. Having a healthy immune system, we know, is very important because, without it, even a small paper cut or a bruise after falling could become life-threatening.

Last, but by no means least, was the reproductive system, the system with the irreplaceable job of bringing new life into this world! We got to learn more about the male and female reproductive systems, showing how they work together to ensure the survival of the human race. This visit reminded me once again about the significance of sexual health education.

We've observed that, when all parts of the body cooperate, they can support one's health and life almost without any problems at all. Thanks for staying by my side during this wonderful adventure. I hope you found out something new about our fantastic anatomy. Keep being inquisitive and continue exploring various aspects of the human body!

THANKS FOR READING

Dear reader,

Thank you for reading *A Guided Tour Through the Human Anatomy*.

If you enjoyed this book, please leave a review where you bought it. It helps more than most people think.

Don't forget your FREE book!

You will also be among the first to know of FREE review copies, discount offers, bonus content, and more.

Go to:

www.SFNonfictionBooks.com

Thanks again for your support.

AUTHOR RECOMMENDATIONS

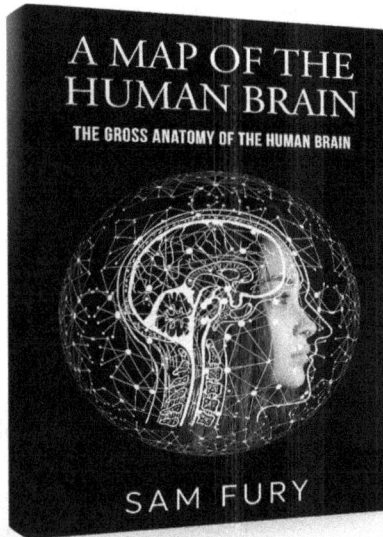

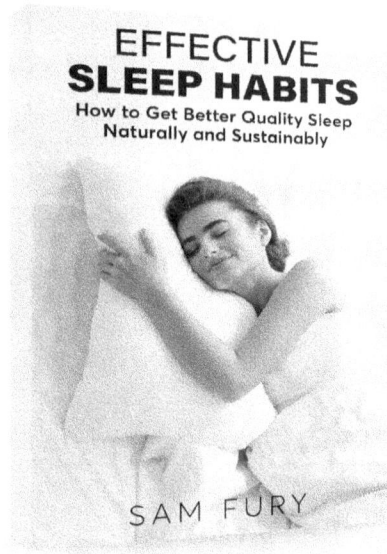

EFFECTIVE
SLEEP HABITS
How to Get Better Quality Sleep
Naturally and Sustainably

SAM FURY

This is the Only Wilderness Medicine Book You Need

Discover what you need to heal yourself, because a little knowledge goes a long way.

Get it now.

www.SFNonfictionbooks.com/Effective-Sleep-Habits

ABOUT SAM FURY

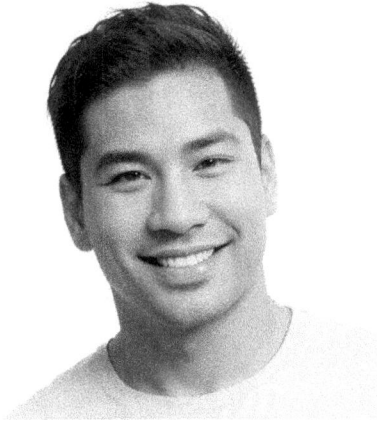

www.SamFury.com

Sam Fury has had a passion for survival, evasion, resistance, and escape (SERE) training since he was a young boy growing up in Australia.

This led him to years of training and career experience in related subjects, including martial arts, military training, and outdoor pursuits.

These days, he spends his time refining his skills and sharing what he learns via his books and blog.

amazon.com/stores/Sam-Fury/author/B00C8Z4U8S

facebook.com/SamFuryOfficial

instagram.com/samfuryofficial

youtube.com/@SamFuryOfficial

x.com/Samfuryoriginal

tiktok.com/@samfuryofficial

REFERENCES

Alexander-Pye, W. (2016, November 21). *Life with dementia: my family's experience.* Alzheimer's Research UK. https://www.alzheimersre searchuk.org/news/life-with-dementia-my-familys-experience/ #author

Bolen, B. (2015, February). *10 interesting facts about your digestive system.* Verywell Health; Verywell Health. https://www.verywellhealth. com/digestive-system-facts-1944708

Byram Healthcare. (2019, April 23). Byram Healthcare. https://www. byramhealthcare.com/blogs/everything-you-should-know-about- the-urinary-system

Cirino, E. (2019, August 5). *11 fun facts about the nervous system.* Healthline. https://www.healthline.com/health/fun-facts-about- the-nervous-system#1

Cleveland Clinic. (2021, September 29). *Muscle.* Cleveland Clinic. https://my.clevelandclinic.org/health/body/21887-muscle

History of the skeleton. (2019). Stanford.edu; Early Science Lab. https://web.stanford.edu/class/history13/earlysciencelab/body/ skeletonpages/skeleton.html

Pulmonary Associates. (2017, April 7). *Lung facts.* Pulmonary Associates of Brandon. https://floridachest.com/pulmonary-blog/ lung-facts

Reproductive system disorders. (n.d.). National Institute of Environmental Health Sciences. https://www.niehs.nih.gov/research/supported/ health/reproductive